RA SEKHI

KEMETIC REIKI

Level One

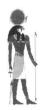
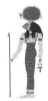

THIS IS A SACRED SYSTEM AND SHOULD BE GUARDED AS SUCH

ABOVE ALL TO YOUR OWN SELF BE TRUE

HONOR THE RA SEKHI SYSTEM

~REKHIT KAJARA ASSATA NEBTHET~

MASTER TEACHER & QUEEN MOTHER OF

RA SEKHI ARTS TEMPLE OF HEALING

I dedicate this work to my youth who are my motivation and inspiration for this work and all that I do.

Also to my Sister Mama Joyce Branch. A true Warrior Healer Priestess Moon Goddess it was a blessing and honor to have you in my life.

We will be calling on you Sister J.

Table of Contents

Foreward 4

History of RA Sekhi 6

Foundations of RA Sekhi 9

Attributes of MAAT 12

Dietary Practices 23

Breathing techniques 25

Energy 27

Aura 34

Aritu/chakras 36

Spirit Guides 43

SEKHMET 45

Colors 67

Hand positions 69

Self treatment positions 75

Symbols 77

Ra Sekhi Principles 81

Ascension 84

Testimonials 87

Afterword 90

Foreward

We are confronted with the energy of the creator every moment of our existence. If you were to survey the earth, what man has created is only an inkling of the what divine energy created billions of years ago and all the wonders are still with us today; the mountains, the oceans, every leafy green being, the soil, the sand, the air and the billions of mankind in our midst. Taking into account this sustenance, these manifestations of nature, they all have ONE thing in common and that is the energy that created and maintains their life.

How does energy work in your life? Let's look at the undeniable ways you know best in this physical realm. You taste energy in the foods you eat and the water you drink. You see energy in the motion of the ocean waves and how your garden grows. You hear energy in the bird's chirps at dawn and the voices of those in your midst. You feel energy with the caress of a summer breeze through your window and the touch of your loved one's gentle hug. You gather the scents of energy as you walk the forest path in spring and from the breath of freshness along the ocean shore. So these things you know...however Universal Energy in the form of truth takes you to a discovery of that which you may not know.

This Universal Energy is; all knowing, all powerful, all wealthy, all forgiving, all beautiful and known to those who have their spiritual eyes open to see what Energy can do within and without. These too are the wise among us, the ones who have activated their divine potential to know and live in the essence of divine energy.

When Alkebulan(*Africa*) was at its best, the sacred spiritual sciences of Kemet(*Egypt*) set forth the divine example of what it is like to live as a mortal god known as Man. The spiritual precepts required a life time of study and daily living of that which is divine. These teachings have begun to be disseminated to the truth seekers in the West, the ones who are to resurrect Amenta to the consciousness of the world. This world of phenomenon exists beyond the ordinary man's consciousness. These realms of existence are exclusively in the spiritual spheres of man which encompass five spiritual senses. These spiritual senses are always activated, but often dormant in the spiritually blind. The first spiritual sense which we give the Kemetic name Ba, supplies and regulates your share of divine energy for your life time in this physical realm. The second spiritual sense called Khu, takes care of your thoughts to remind you of your divine connection. The third spiritual sense, Khat, concerns itself with the flow of the physical body to ensure you master procreation. The fourth spiritual sense, Ka, activates your emotional/physical sense's guide to ensure that you enjoy this physical life while fulfilling divine purpose. Last, your fifth spiritual sense, Sekhem, elevates the wisdom faculty through your life experiences to prepare the soul for the next lifetime. We walk with many eyes to see and many truths to find, "those who seek spiritual truth are few and only a few of those find it".

THE ENERGY OF THE UNIVERSE IS YOU. The essence of all matter and substance comes from within. When one has connected with the power within, all of the right things happen at the right time, in the right order and for the right reasons. This beautiful existence is only for those who live in the realm of balance created by the knowledge of truth according to divine law.

There is a Kemetic Proverb that says, "If you learn that you ARE the Energy of Life, and that you only happen to be out of the energy at the moment, you will return to that energy and know life." The journey to and through Ra Sekhi is one of the roads to KNOW LIFE.

-Dr. Akua Gray
  Accra, Ghana
  August 25, 2012

HISTORY AND PURPOSE OF RA SEKHI

All sciences including the healing arts were practiced and mastered in ancient Kemet. The evidence of this work was left on the walls of the pyramids to stand the test of time. They also stand as a testimony of truth of our intelligence and development long before other nations existed. There are pictures and stories of healing rites, using symbols and the hands as healing tools. Life force and chakras were mentioned in the pyramid texts as well as mantras or hekau (words of power). The use of crystals, plants, metals, water, animals and other forces of nature were also used. What is now called reiki has been practiced by healers and priests in Kemet thousands of years before it was renamed reiki.

Great healers from all over the world were known to have gone to Kemet or Ancient Egypt to learn and study with the masters of healing and higher consciousness. The work of our ancient masters has continued in different countries, by healers all over the world. It continues now though this and many other healing movements going on right now, for the purpose of healing and restoring MAAT to the Earth once again.

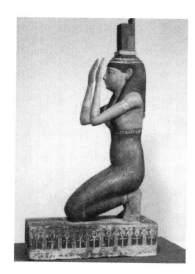

Self Healing

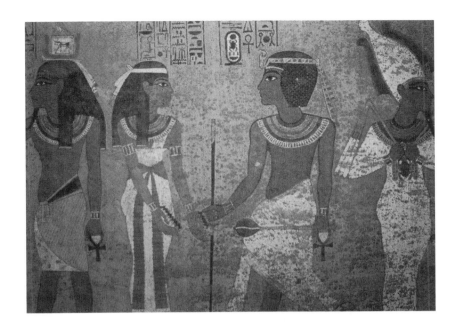

Notice the energy flowing from the Goddess hands.
The wavy lines are called nini or nu and refers to the
energy that flows from our hands.

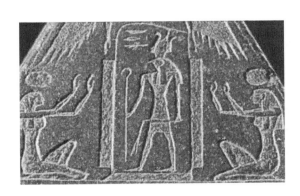

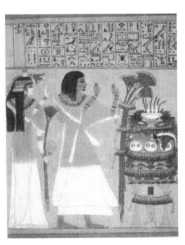

There are pictures of hands being used to give and
receive energy found in pyramids all over Kemet.

The Rebirth

My path to healing began at sixteen years of age when I was diagnosed with a painful and so-called incurable disease. The pain became so overwhelming one day, and I was led to place my hands where I felt pain and to pray. I prayed to THE CRETOR using all the names for God I had heard of, as well as angels to come and heal me. The next day the pain was gone and it never came back. It wasn't until the year 2000 when I read about reiki that I realized I had used the same technique on myself years ago. I was attuned in Level I, II, and the Master Level in Tibetan reiki by Rayys Sekhem of Brooklyn, NY in 2000. During this time I was also a student of Queen Afua and began facilitating grassroots Sacred Woman circles. This was my introduction to GODDESS SEKHMET as well as other powerful NTRU, Gods and Goddess of Ancient Kemet.

As my work continued, my relationship with Sekhmet grew. I began to receive messages saying I should teach reiki to my people and give the proper credit of the practice to our Kemetic ancestors. I was told that all science has its roots in the Nile Valley region, known as Kemet. They left proof on the walls of the pyramids and in ancient texts. This knowledge and the healing traditions left on the walls of the pyramids should be shared with our community, using our own symbols, sounds, and tools.

The name RA SEKHI came through and this healing practice was reborn. Since this healing modality was reborn in 2007, we attuned over 100 practitioners in over 10 states. GODDESS SEKHMET says that the more of us who overstand how to use our energy for healing, the sooner we will see healing and MAAT manifest in our community. The more of us who call on her, the sooner we will see MAAT on this realm once again.

I am also a certified Afrikan Wholistic Health Consultant, Traditional Afrikan High Priestess, Heal Thyself Ambassador of Wellness, Natural Healer, Artist, Activist, Educator and Mother.

I have taught Black History, Art, music, health, PE, yoga, womb wisdom and Ra Sekhi to hundreds of all ages for over fifteen years, throughout the Midwest, east coast, and southern US. I have dedicated my life to promote health and wellness and to uplift my people.

The purpose of RA SEKHI being reborn at this time is to bring Divine healing to people of Afrikan descent. We believe we can heal the spiritual, emotional, mental, and physical ills that have plagued our community by tapping into THE POWER OF THE DIVINE UNLIMITED LIGHT FORCE to heal and reshape our community. With the help of our Ancestors, Spirit Guides, Deities and Light Forces, hard work, and diligence, we know that THE POWER IS IN OUR HANDS to manifest this for the betterment of ourselves, our families, our community, and OUR WORLD. ASE. May it be so.

AMEN RA , MAAT

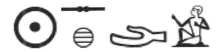

FOUNDATIONS OF RA SEKHI

RA SEKHI is based on the ancient energy healing systems of our ancestors in Kemet and throughout Afrika. It is a wholistic healing technique which uses energy to manipulate and balance the physical, emotional, mental and spiritual bodies. It works to create positive changes in ones energy fields to bring healing and relief to dis-eases of all kinds. It uses the power and energy of RA/RAAT, THE CREATOR AND CREATRESS, THE SUPREME LIGHT BEINGS WHO ARE THE DIVINE LIVING ENERGY MOVING THROUGHOUT AND ANIMATING ALL OF THEIR CREATED ENTITIES IN CREATION. THEY ARE THE GREAT SPIRIT WHO OPERATE AND SHARE THEIR ENERGY AND POWER THROUGH THE SUN, ATEN. They share light and energy with all constantly and their source is infinite .

The word sekhi means to play, to overthrow, to beat a drum, to strike a light, to kindle a fire. This refers to the vibration, energy and life force that we use in our healing work. RA SEKHI uses Sekhem, also called Chi or Ki, which is the life force energy that emanates from within all living things. Sekhem enlivens and sustains all of creation. It lies dormant within every human being until it is activated and elevated through prayer, meditation, yoga, dance, initiation, ritual or other spiritual work. Our Sekhem connects us to THE GODDESS SEKHMET, THE GREAT HEALER, THE DESTROYER OF EVIL, GODDESS OF MENSTRUATION , WHOSE NAME MEANS POWERFUL. SEKHMET IS THE MOTHER AND HEAD DEITY OF RA SEKHI. SHE GIVES THE POWER TO PASS AND CONNECT OUR SEKHEM WITH RA/RAAT. It is through her that this Divine system has been reborn. As we call on her more, we can break destructive cycles that lead to dis-ease. She is known to restore Maat when there is chaos.

RA SEKHI consciously and actively connects the energy of RA/RAAT with ones own Sekhem to channel, radiate and harmonize sending healing energy within and to another. The healer or channel should be of pure heart, body, mind and spirit for the energy to flow as intended. It is through Spiritual work, attunement or initiation that this process begins for the healer.

Our ancestors treated healing as well as everything else in life wholistically. They would appeal to all senses to bring MAAT, healing and projection of energy. Therefore RA SEKHI reminds us to use our hands, our thoughts, prayers, mantras/hekau, crystals, colors, symbols, aromatherapy, and other natural medicine and tools for healing. It is through the use of natural tools that healing energy is shared to balance the mental, spiritual, emotional and physical bodies. We use RA SEKHI to bring MAAT to the root of dis-ease to balance and heal the issues that have not been resolved from this and other lifetimes. RA SEKHI is similar to what is called laying on of hands and has been a part of many ritual and healing practices from Kemet, through South and West Afrika and into Amerika during enslavement. The ashe or spiritual power is received through ancestral and blood transmission: it is inborn in those whose destiny and gift is healing. We use our connection to the higher forces or deities (Neteru, Orisha, Abosom, Lwa, etc...) to channel light energy. The practice of laying hands has been used by "juju" people in the backwoods of the north and south. It is used through seers, those who practice divination, herbal remedies, aromatherapy and others who practice ancestral traditions. It is used in churches when people get possessed or are guided to lay their hands and pray over someone. It is used by mothers when their child gets a cut and mama kisses it and makes it better. All of these examples share one key element that is the core of energy healing intention. When your Spirit is strong your intention will make your work stronger and successful, it will work as you intend it to.

When practicing RA SEKHI it is important to have a general overstanding of the body, the organs, the Aritu/chakras and meridians as well as how energy effects them. This will allow you to use your tools to balance and harmonize the entire system. As a practitioner it is key to have proper eating habits, cleansing of body, mind and spirit, exercise, fasting, spiritual development, and proper rest. This will assist in your purification process, attaining higher consciousness, a light heart and a high vibration. The healer/channel should be of pure heart, body, mind and spirit for the energy to flow as it is intended. It is through Spiritual work, attunement or initiation that this process elevates for the healer. The RA Sekhi attunement is a passing of energy from the teacher to the initiate. It will begin a detoxing process in your life to assist you with being in alignment with your higher self and to restore MAAT in all aspects of your life. This process can take weeks, months or years, depending on the work that you do for yourself. As well as the time and energy you give towards healing yourself.

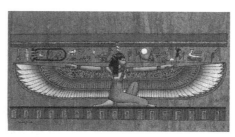

Goddess MAAT

The observance of the 42 principles of MAAT are part of the path of RA SEKHI practice. These laws were left in the pyramid texts thousands of years ago. One should recite the principle of MAAT daily to encode them in your mind. These Divine guidelines have been used in societies where police were not necessary because everyone overstood basic moral laws. Now those of us who use them can remind others with our example in how we should live and behave. We also observe the attributes of MAAT, which are universal laws, listed below.

7 Attributes of MAAT

ORDER

The first virtue is order because it is the first thing that comes out of the creative process, nothing is possible without order. There is the cosmic order, the natural order of living things, the social order of man and woman, personal order, and the spiritual order of humanity. Our ancestors lived in harmony with nature and had a natural order to their day to day activities. MAAT shows us that we must have order in the way we think, the way we keep our homes, the way we eat, dress, handle our business, etc. When you have your life in order you are on time and flow with the natural order of time.

BALANCE

It is the state of a system that is in equilibrium at any given moment. It is the noble aspiration of an individual seeking and sustaining in all behavior, speech and thought the "middle way". There should be balance in how you manage your time and energy. There should be time to develop the mind, the body and the spirit. There should be time to work, rest and relax or play. There should be balance in our time for self, time for friends and time for family. There should be balance in the amount of time we spend in front of the TV or computer and the amount of time we spend in nature. Seek to create and maintain balance in all aspects of your life.

HARMONY

It comes from having order and balance in your life. It is the state of peace which one feels when out in nature, left undisturbed my man. It deals with the vibration and flow of things. When one is in harmony they feel a certain peace and joy, regardless of what is going on in the world around them. They remain calm in the midst of storm. They learn to flow with the ups and downs of life, knowing that all is in Divine order at all times, even if it doesn't feel like it. It is associated with beauty, joy and peace. We seek to have harmony in our work, in our relationships, in our homes and all aspects of our lives.

PROPRIETY/COMPASSION

The most universal human desire is for love, happiness, affection and the avoidance of suffering, these feelings develop compassion. Other qualities of compassion are empathy, kindness, and patience. Acts of compassion are helping the weak, hungry, sick, and caring for others that you may or may not know. Sharing a smile, hug or kind words can make a huge difference in one's life. Have compassion in the way you deal with yourself, with others, with animals, plants and all of nature.

RECIPROCITY

It defines forms of exchange, the movement of energy, goods and services from one to another. It promotes mutual obliga-tion in emotional, material, psychological and spiritual areas of experience between man and woman, children and extended family, friends, the community and elders. It is associated with complementary accountability and gratitude. Simply put, eve-rything you do comes back to you. Every thought, word, and action echo's in the universe and will bring the energy you put out right back. This works regardless if it is positive or negative energy you put out. Every thing is created with a thought, then the words, then it is manifested on the physical plane. So watch what you think and say. Remember the saying treat people like you want to be treated. The law of attraction is within MAAT. It is also called karma.

TRUTH

It is defined by facts, experiences, observation and perspec-tive. It is absolute and timeless. It is consciousness and one must speak and live truth. Be true to yourself. Be true to your purpose in life. Know your limits, know what you need to focus on. You have to know yourself to know what is true for you. Know and respect that what is true for you is not always true for others. Yet there are universal truths that are true for every-one. Qualities of truth are openness, authenticity, honesty and trust.

RIGHTEOUSNESS/JUSTICE

It is the goal of the initiate to live with social, economic and political rightness. Qualities include, fairness, flexibility and just doing what is right, virtuous and morally right. Living with righteousness is about having a good heart. Doing what is best for yourself and others, without bringing hurt and harm to others. It is not religion that makes one righteous, there are positive and negative ones in every religion. It is the heart of the person, their words and actions that reflect if one is righteous.

THE 42 DECLARATION OF RIGHTEOUSNESS

1. *I WILL NOT DO WRONG*
2. *I WILL NOT STEAL*
3. *I WILL NOT ACT WITH VIOLENCE*
4. *I WILL NOT KILL*
5. *I WILL NOT BE UNJUST*
6. *I WILL NOT CAUSE PAIN*
7. *I WILL NOT WASTE FOOD*
8. *I WILL NOT LIE*
9. *I WILL NOT DESECRATE HOLY PLACES*
10. *I WILL NOT SPEAK EVIL*
11. *I WILL NOT ABUSE MY SEXUALITY*
12. *I WILL NOT CAUSE THE SHEDDING OF TEARS*
13. *I WILL NOT SOW SEEDS OF REGRET*
14. *I WILL NOT BE AN AGGRESSOR*
15. *I WILL NOT ACT GUILOEFULLY*
16. *I WILL NOT LAY WASTE THE PLOWED LAND*
17. *I WILL NOT BEAR FALSE WITNESS*
18. *I WILL NOT SET MY MOUTH IN MOTION(AGAINST ANY PERSON)*
19. *I WILL NOT BE WRATHFUL AND ANGRY EXCEPT FOR A JUST CAUSE*
20. *I WILL NOT COPULATE WITH A MAN'S WIFE*

21. I WILL NOT COPULATE WITH A WOMAN'S HUSBAND
22. I WILL NOT POLLUTE MYSELF
23. I WILL NOT CAUSE TERROR
24. I WILL NOT POLLUTE THE EARTH
25. I WILL NOT SPEAK IN ANGER
26. I WILL NOT TURN FROM WORDS OF RIGHT AND TRUTH
27. I WILL NOT UTTER CURSES
28. I WILL NOT INITIATE A QUARREL
29. I WILL NOT BE EXCITABLE OR CONTENTIOUS
30. I WILL NOT BE PREJUSICE
31. I WILL NOT BE AN EAVESDROPPER
32. I WILL NOT SPEAK OVERMUCH
33. I WILL NOT COMMIT TREASON AGAINST MY ANCESTORS
34. I WILL NOT WASTE WATER
35. I WILL NOT DO EVIL
36. I WILL NOT BE ARROGANT
37. I WILL NOT BLASPHEME NTR (THE ONE MOST HIGH)
38. I WILL NOT COMMIT FRAUD
39. I WILL NOT DEFRAUD TEMPLE OFFERINGS
40. I WILL NOT PLUNDER THE DEAD
41. I WILL NOT MISTREAT CHILDREN
42. I WILL NOT MISTREAT ANIMALS

These Laws of MAAT are also known as the Declaration of Innocence. They are drawn from the "Pert Em HRU" (the Book of Coming Forth by Day) the oldest Afrikan book of Holy Scriptures. With these laws our Ancient Ancestors maintained a society without policemen for thousands of years. In the early morning say "I will not..." In the evening say "I have not..." This is our mental inventory.

This translation from Sen-Ur Hru Ankh Ra Semaj se Ptah High Priest of The Shrine of Ptah.

The laws should be said everyday to assist you in maintaining MAAT. You can also meditate on one principle per day with your family to introduce and promote MAAT in your home.

MAAT teaches us to keep our hearts light, how to treat each other, ourselves and the world. We must also bring MAAT to our past. This is the work of lightening the heart. One can go back through their memory and consider each situation that caused anger or sadness and then truly reassess the situation. Cry, scream, shout, or write letters about your feelings. This will help release the pain. Then look for the lessons, look at the fact that if you had not come through this situation you would not be where you are today. Find the blessings so that you will stop seeing it as a bad situation. It may be hard but this is part of the process. Take as much time as you need.

Then we must also go through the process of forgiving. Forgive yourself for allowing you to hurt or be hurt. Forgive yourself for hurting others and ask for this cycle to stop. Then you must also forgive others for hurting you. Forgiving them does not mean to forget what they have done. It does not mean to put yourself in the place to allow them to hurt you again. However it does mean that you do not allow negative low vibration emotions continue to dwell in your body temple. That is the point, to release the sadness, anger, fear, worry, and doubt because these negative emotions feed and attract more negativity into your life.

When your heart is light you can be at peace with your life and all of the ups and downs in between. That is when you can say that all is in divine order. Even the things we don't have an understanding of, they are still part of the order of the universe and are a reflection of the time that we are living in. We must remember that we only have control of ourselves and doing the best we can do, is the best we can do. As each individual begins to change and heal we will see the positive changes in our community that we want to see.

When you truly forgive, you can talk about a situation with no emotion at all. When your heart is light you will attract the blessings and goodness of life to you. In our community, we've had so many years of trauma and strife that we continue to attract it to us. When we break the cycle of negative thinking patterns and habits, we will receive overall health and wellness in every aspect of our lives.

These Liberation prayers will help to free you from the energetic ties that may be blocking your vibration. They will work to clear your heart as well. It is good to say them once a day for seven days, or let your Spirit guide.

Liberation Prayers

1. Prayer of Liberation:

For anyone whom I have knowingly or unknowingly hurt in my lifetime.

I sincerely pray for all the individuals whom I have knowingly or unknowingly hurt in my life.

I ask that the content and energy of this prayer will be used to comfort, educate and liberate anyone whom I am guilty of hurting.

I ask that this prayer energy will heal them of any resentment and pain that they bear because of me. I am sincerely sorry.

I realize that it is only when I have made amends (whenever possible, directly) to all those whom I have hurt, that I can be truly forgiven of my wrongs and released from accusation on earth and in the spirit world.

I further realize that genuine repentance and forgiveness are manifested only:

By apologizing for my past wrong doings, when possible and/or appropriate.

By not repeating the same wrongs

And by endeavoring to do only good in my thoughts, words and actions.

Lead me to overcome all that is not in accordance with your will, Heavenly Father.

2. Prayer of forgiveness and liberation:

For anyone who has knowingly or unknowingly hurt me.

I sincerely and unconditionally forgive all those who have hurt me during their lifetime on earth or in the spirit world.

I willingly surrender my negative thoughts and feelings towards them so that I may be set free and be able to grow in forgiveness and love.

Only by letting go of all my resentments and by forgiving and loving unconditionally will I be able to complete my own spiritual growth toward God.

I pray that those people who have hurt me, will be liberated through my forgiving them, so that they, too, may be free to grow in love and fulfill their purpose.

3. Prayer of liberation:

For anyone on earth or in the spirit world whom my ancestors have knowingly or unknowingly hurt.

Because my ancestors do not have the energy in the spirit world to grow easily by directly making amends for their wrongs, I, being still on earth and having that necessary energy, must take responsibility to help liberate them of accusation from sin so they can be free to grow higher and become one with our Heavenly Father.

I realize that I am a descendant of my ancestry and that I - through spiritual inheritance - bear a portion of responsibility for my ancestors' sins.

Unless they are liberated, I and my family cannot be free from accusation, and thus temptation and invasion from the negative spirit world, nor be free to totally become one with our Heavenly Father.

I realize that I am taking responsibility for my ancestors' sins by praying for any and all people who are on earth or in the spirit world whom my ancestors are guilty of hurting.

I sincerely pray for all the people whom my ancestors in the spirit world knowingly or unknowingly hurt during their earthly lifetime.

I ask that the content and energy of my prayers - on behalf of my ancestors - go to these people to comfort, educate and liberate them.

I ask that this prayer will heal them of any negative thoughts or feelings that they bear because of my ancestors. I am sincerely sorry and apologize on behalf of my ancestors.

4. Prayer of liberation:

For my ancestors in the spirit world for whom I am providentially responsible:

I sincerely pray for all my ancestors for whom I am providentially responsible.

I ask that the content and energy of this prayer be used to educate and liberate my ancestors who are guilty of doing wrongs against Your Will, Heavenly Father.

I ask that through this prayer, my ancestors may be forgiven of the sins they committed while on earth as I vicariously repent for them.

I am deeply sorry for their actions not in accordance with your Divine Will, Heavenly Father and I apologize for them on their behalf. Please forgive them.

I also lovingly admonish my ancestors to:

"Give up all negative thoughts and feelings by forgiving everyone who hurt you while you were on earth."

"Only by forgiving and thus giving up your negative state of mind will you be able to grow in the spirit world."

"Hear this prayer and gain understanding."

"Apply what I am telling you and you will find yourself gradually ascending into a higher level of existence in the spirit world."

"Serve your descendants and proper others on earth and in the spirit world with a loving and grateful heart and you will most easily and quickly overcome your negative, self-inhibiting thoughts and feelings."

Ra Sekhi is an Afrikan centered healing system. Therefore part of our work involves reprogramming the way we think, speak, act and live. We have been raised in a culture that is quite different from our own. As we work to restore MAAT in our lives we must accept our traditional culture, ways and behavior. This is first step in our healing journey. Our ancestors had very high morals and standards, as well as particular ways of dealing with family, relationships, etc. As we do the work to heal ourselves if should create a trickling effect that spreads to our family and all that we are connected to.

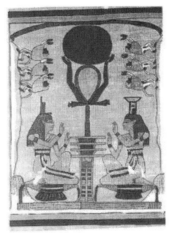

Auset and Nebthet working with life force

The chart on the following page is helpful in the restoration of our culture and way.

The history of humanity will remain confused as long as we fail to distinguish between the two cradles, in which nature fashioned the instincts, temperaments, habits, and ethical concepts of the two subdivisions, before they met each other, after a long separation, dating back to prehistoric times."

Cheikh Anta Diop

A COMPARATIVE STUDY OF DIOP'S "TWO CRADLES" THEORY

AFRIKAN	EUROPEAN
UNDERSTAND CREATOR AS GOOD	VIEW GOD AS EVIL
ARE ONE WITH NATURE	NEED TO CONTROL NATURE
GROUPNESS, A WAY OF LIFE	INDIVIDUALISM, THE SUPREME VIRTUE
LIVE INTERPERSONAL INTER-DEPENDENCE	ADVOCATE PERSONAL INDEPEND-ENCE
FOCUS ON FAMILY LOVE	SELF-CENTERED
COOPERATION, A WAY OF LIFE	COMPETITION A WAY OF LIFE
GENTLENESS AND PEACEFUL	CRUELTY AND AGGRESSIVENESS
DECISIONS BY MORAL RIGHT-EOUSNESS	DECISIONS OF POLITICAL EXPEDI-ENCY
PRACTICE COLLECTIVE RE-SPONSIBILITY	ADVOCATE PERSONAL RESPONSI-BILITY
FOCUS ON SAMENESS/ SIMILARITY	FOCUS ON UNIQUENESS/ DIFFERENCE
SPIRITUAL ORIENTATION	MATERIALISTIC ORIENTATION
RESPECT IS NATURAL TO BE-ING	MUST EARN RESPECT
PRACTICE GENDER EQUALITY	PRACTICE MALE SUPERIORITY
LOVE FOR STRANGERS	FEAR OF STRANGERS
SIBLING RESPONSIBILITY	SIBLING RIVALRY
OPTIMISTIC WORLDVIEW	PESSIMISTIC WORLDVIEW
SEDENTARY	NOMADIC
NO NOTION OF ORIGINAL SIN	ORIGINAL SIN BLAMED ON FE-MALE
SPIRITUAL SURVIVAL, THE UL-TIMATE	PHYSICAL SURVIVAL, THE ULTI-MATE
NO FEAR, GUILT, SHAME IN SPIRITUALITY	FEAR, GUILT, SHAME IN RELIGION
LAW BASED ON TRUTH AND JUSTICE	LAW BASED ON DECEPTION, CON-TROL
EQUALITY IN HUMANITY	WHITE SUPREMACY

Dietary Practices

While on your healing journey you will want to eat the best food that you can eat. This will feed and nourish your cells and organs promoting overall health and wellness in your body. It is important to consume the least amount of pollutant as possible. Reducing the amount preservatives, preservatives and gmo food is key. Eat more raw fruits and vegetables. Take time to learn about proper eating and herbs. Remember that what you consume feeds and fuels your blood, your brain and your organs. Eat high quality organic foods. The money you invest in eating healthy now will save you money in hospital bills and prescriptions later.

* Avoid junk food and fast food

* Avoid white sugar, white flour and other white products that have been bleached of the nutrients

* Avoid meat and dairy products

* Avoid GMO food (genetically modified foods like seedless fruit)

* Avoid colored sugar water, soda, fruit drinks, etc.

* Avoid processed meat substitutes

* Eat plenty fresh vegetables, fruits, grains, nuts and seeds

* Eat a green salad everyday

* Use fresh herbs in tea and your meals

We also suggest that you take time to clean your body of toxins that have built up from years of eating poor food. This process can take from 3 months to 3 years. I went through a cleansing process for two years, fasting for 21 days at a time, also doing enemas and taking herbal remedies to assist this process. When you are full of toxins you may have symptoms like constipation, headaches, indigestion, insomnia, congestion, etc. These are signs your body is giving you to pay attention to yourself. The tradition way to relieve the body of these symptoms is to fast and cleanse using herbs and water.

It is said that each year we should fast 1 day for every year we have lived. So a 40 year old would fast for 40 days in that year. This is done to help maintain balance in the body. there are many ways to fast. You can fast from cooked food (raw food fast), fast from eating meat. You can do a water fast (drink water only) , a juice fast, a fruit fast, etc. The point is to gain discipline and self control while giving the body an opportunity to rest and purify itself. Fasting also promotes spiritual development and can be seen as a way of making a sacrifice of the self. It is a part of our culture to cleanse and purify our bodies and spirits this way. It is important to maintain a high vibration and for overall wellness.

Set a cycle for yourself and your family. You can fast one day a week for 24 hours just drink juice, tea and water. As an alternative you can do a longer fast around the changing of the seasons, the equinox or solstice times. Fast for 7 to 21 days or more this will help prevent you from getting sick in the upcoming season and will also put you in tune with the earth as she goes through her shifting process. Make sure to take herbal remedies to clear the colon, kidneys, liver, blood, etc. Also a series of enemas and colonics are important in the cleansing process. You will be surprised how much waste the average person walks around with. Our goal is to be have a light heart and light and healthy body.

You may want to set some time aside to focus on your self healing process. After going through level 1 we ask everyone to take 21 days to focus on doing the work on themselves. This is an excellent addition to your healing journey. It will give you the opportunity to begin to incorporate Ra Sekhi into your lifestyle.

BREATHING TECHNIQUES

The importance of breathing can be highlighted by stating that it is the gift of life. Have you ever been nervous and took a deep breath to settle your spirit? Do you remember being upset and hearing momma or grandmama tell you to slow down and take deep breaths? Women, do you remember giving birth and being told to breathe through the contractions? Do you remember the last time you stepped outside and took a deep breath of the fresh spring air? Breath helps to regulate our emotions and it brings fresh oxygen to our body system. Without the breath, we have no life. Our Sekhem, life force, flows through our breath and our blood. So we must be conscious of our breath.

To cultivate our sekhem we should practice conscious breathing everyday. Yoga, Afrikan dance, tai chi, qi gong, martial arts and other exercise is important to keep your energy and sekhem strong.

What is proper breathing?

Proper breathing is done when the diaphragm expands causing the stomach to expand. When you exhale, you are relaxing the diaphragm and contracting the stomach. Best breathing is done when spine is straight allowing for the vital organs to get the oxygen they need.

These are some conscious breathing techniques that we use.

Deep Breathing: Deep breathing is done by breathing in through your nose and out through the mouth. This breath is slow and deep. While breathing in through your nose you can count mentally. If you are a person who has never focused on their breathing before, counting to four is a good way to begin. Once you have inhaled, you need to hold the breath for the same count. To release the breath, release through the mouth for a count of four. Practice deep breathing everyday and increase your count with your practice.

Alternate Nostril Breathing

This helps to balance the right and left side of the brain. The right side controls the left side of the body while the left side controls the right side of the body. You begin by placing your thumb on the right nostril and breathing in deep through the left nostril for a count of four. Next you use your index or pinky finger to close your left nostril. Keep both nostrils pinched and hold the breath for a count of four. Next release the right nostril, breath in for a count of four, pinch off both nostrils and hold for a count of four, release the left nostril and begin the process all over again. Remember to alternate breathing in the right nostril and out the left.

Fire Breathing

Fire breathing helps to raise the Sekhem (Life Force Energy). It is the process of rapid breathing. The process of breathing is similar to the deep breathing in the concept that you are filling up the abdomen and releasing the breath fully by contracting the abdomen, breathing in and out of the nose. However in this case, you are NOT holding the breath but you are breathing at a very rapid pace. A beginner should start by doing this 30-50 times. If you become light headed or begin hyperventilating, breathe into a small PAPER bag to restore you carbon balance. Once you have mastered fire breathing, you will find that you can increase your numbers to the thousands without experiencing light headedness.

Each of these methods can be used to assist you before beginning a healing session. Conscious breathing will help you center and ground yourself. Breathe before you begin your meditations, before doing spiritual work or just to relax yourself. Conscious breathing should be done daily to maintain high vitality.

ABOUT ENERGY

Energy is the unseen force that is in all living things. Energy cannot be created or destroyed, it just is. Energy is in the sun, moon, stars, the Earth, water and everything living. It flows around and within us. It vibrates through colors, sound, symbols and all things living. As humans, it surrounds us and moves through us via our blood and our breath. Our energy moves through us in patterns of vibration, also called energy fields, in the same way that a song moves through patterns of energetic vibrations. So therefore if our energy vibration is high, the energy we consume is high, the energy we attract, what we think and speak has a high vibration as well. Our energy is primarily fed through our thoughts, what we consume and our environment. However all things that affect our senses also affect our energy and our vibration.

Our personal energy is called our life force. It is connected to our breath, blood and our spirit and leaves our body when we make our transition. It continues to be a part of the all, the universal energy that sustains us all. Our life force energy is called sekhem, prana, chi or ki. Most of us are unaware of this energy and therefore don't ever reach our greatest potential. Those who become aware of it and learn to control it can do things such as break a stack of bricks, overcome any obstacles, astral travel, manifest things, etc. There are many techniques available for cultivating sekhem. Meditating, doing yoga, tai chi, chi gong or other martial arts share valuable lessons on developing and building sekhem/chi.

Our sekhem is connected to our will, our drive to live and our motivation to get things done. So when our energy is high we have the ability to do what we need to do in a timely fashion.

When we are behind in our work or find ourselves procrastinating it is associated with low vitality and is associated with how we feel, how we are thinking, etc. We have to consciously do things to keep our sekhem balanced, strong and with a high vibration. Remember that everything that affects your senses affects your energy, your sekhem. Things that you see, hear, smell, taste, touch and feel can bring your vibration up or down. This is why we eat sweets though we know it is not good for our bodies; it is sweet and good for our spirit. It can make you feel good and raise your energy because it tastes good, have it now and then as a treat, because overall too much chocolate can cause problems in your physical body which will lower your vibration.

When we go through good experiences it is good for our energy, it raises our vibration. When we go through traumatic experiences it creates negative vibrations, our energy level decreases and our energy field changes. If we go through several traumatic experiences, our energy field can build layers of unbalanced energy. For example black women who have gone through lifetimes of traumatic experiences create children who are born with layers of negative energy fields. So we come back to the Earth with energy that was not healed and processed in previous lifetimes which can lead to negative behavior patterns, poor character, negative thinking habits, and so on.

We come here at this time with the opportunity to bring these things, our energy (inner chi) into balance. We have a chance to correct our mistakes, learn our lessons, raise our vibrations and experience the ascension of our souls. We come to correct ourselves and make ourselves more perfect, or Godly. It is up to every individual to find their mission in life, their purpose and to fulfill it to the best of their ability. It is also up to everyone to see their shortcomings, to learn their lessons and to live in MAAT, or with good character. That is the God force, the Goddess within us that we all come here with. We are made in the image and likeness of the Goddess and that gives us the power and energy to manifest all things. When we are aware that our energy is universal and infinite we know we are connected to the all. Our abilities and possibilities become unlimited.

Our connection to the infinite source gives us the ability to create our lives the way that we want and live our dreams because that is in alignment with our highest self. It gives us the ability to heal ourselves and to do everything that we desire to have all that we desire all that we need and more. Our thoughts, words, actions and energy create our world. When you understand energy, how to protect and keep your energy high, you can create a better world for yourself. See yourself as a part of the energy flow, a being which absorbs and releases energy constantly. You can choose to take and radiate high or low frequency energy. The high frequency energy includes love, harmony, peace, joy and positive feeling, the lower the frequency the lower the feelings disappointment, doubt; sadness, anger and fear are the lowest. You can tell where your energy is based on high you feel. You can also control or choose how you are going to feel.

The mind controls the way you think and the way you feel. its knowledge or level of consciousness, the ego, thinking patterns, behavior, intentions, imagination, dreams, focus also effect the energy and the sekhem as well as the ability to use sekhem. When the mind, the heart and the will are in agreement then one is balanced and in MAAT. The fruits of being on this energetic vibration are success, joy, physical or financial gains and most importantly peace within. These are people who seem to have it all, not the rich and famous but the ones who have successful businesses or nonprofits; they have beautiful families and seem to be happy and healthy no matter what happens. That is the peace and happiness we all seek to have, that is having heaven on earth.

We have energy that flows within us. As women, it comes up from the earth through our feet and move up through our back to our head and then moves down to our feet and back up again. For men it comes from the heavens through the crown, moves down and back around. You will find that as we get older many of us begin to have problems in our knees and hips, because the energy becomes blocked at these points from us sitting upright in chairs for so many days. That is why it is so important to exercise, to keep the air, the blood and energy flowing through us properly. Any form of dance, all sports, walking, swimming are all excellent ways to keep your energy flowing, your life force strong and keep you healthy overall.

When you drink fresh carrot juice you feel it instantly rejuvenating your body as it flows through your system. Not only because it is liquid and gets in your blood faster, but also fresh juice is still living so it has more vitality, vitamins, minerals and energy then cooked (pasteurized) juices and foods. It is said that eating food that is still attached to the ground is the best way to eat because the food is still fully charged with energy. Foods that are cooked lose their vitamin, mineral and energy levels. So as you see your veggies turning from a bright green to a dull green color it is losing its energy or vitality. So it cannot add very much to your own energy.

Packaged, processed and junk food does not add to your energy, in fact they may lower your energy because they introduce foreign, man-made chemicals into your body. Remember your life force does flow through your blood which also feeds your heart and brain.

You can feel the energy when you go into an environment where there has been chaos or negativity, you can feel the energy in a room when you light a certain incense or say a prayer. You may feel your energy shift when watching television, listening to the radio or being around certain people. Energy can attach itself to you, your thoughts, feelings and/or your aura. You may feel a shift in energy when you aritu or chakras are out of balance. Sometimes you feel a shift in energy and are unaware of what you are really feeling.

In working to keep your vibration high you want to be mindful of the things that you consume because they also affect the energy. Not just the things that you eat but also the things you see, listen to and the people you are around. When you eat foods that are alive, foods that are raw and organic, if possible, you will receive the highest amount of energy from them.

Be mindful of the things you watch, what you read and look at throughout your day. Watching violent or dramatic images will lower your energetic vibration. Most TV programs, advertising, magazines and newspapers work to over stimulate our lower energy. They keep us sad, angry or upset which keeps us from being balanced overall. I have found the same to be true with the music available to us today. When we hear words spoken to us repeatedly every day, it becomes like a chant and begins to influence our psyche and energy fields. Just at the TV and radio works on electric waves for us to see and hear it, those same electric wave patterns affect our own patterns.

There are many traditional ways to balance and harmonize your energy when necessary. Chanting positive affirmations, reading spiritual books, prayer, meditation, exercise, listening to uplifting music, using crystal or oils, eating live and healthy food and spending time in nature are some of the best ways to keep your energy positive and balanced. Many Spiritual people pray throughout the day to help them stay focused and positive. Smiling and staying positive are also helpful in keeping energy balanced..

Spiritual baths are powerful for keeping energy balanced and cleansing the aura. A Spiritual Bath is a powerful healing and balancing experience. It cleans the unseen energy that builds up when going around different people. You know the experience of being around someone angry or sad and after talking to them you feel the same way. This energy can penetrate your emotional, mental, and spiritual body as well as your aura. A spiritual bath is one way to balance and purify yourself.

A spiritual bath becomes Spiritual by adding natural elements, your words of power and intent to the water. Some good things to add; sea or epsom salt, crystals, essential oils, herbs, natural coloring, clear alcohol (rum or gin), florida or rose water, flowers, fruit, milk, etc.... You can make a variety of baths to assist with different things like a protection bath, attraction bath, healing bath, clearing bath, etc....Choose crystals, herbs and colors depending on the properties of the elements to match your needs. Rain, river, and ocean water are powerful additions to spiritual baths as well. They add the energy of movement and magnify the energy of your bath.

It can be made one of two ways :

1. Add the ingredients to a tub of water, soak and immerse yourself in the bath while meditating, chanting or praying, on your purpose for the bath

2. Add the ingredients to a vessel of water it should be made of natural material like glass, wood, ceramic, or calabash. While adding the ingredients meditate, pray and chant your purpose for the bath while mixing the bath with your hands. Wash yourself physically first then pour spiritual bath mixture over you with a smaller natural vessel.

After the bath it is good to dress in white and stay in a meditative state, just relax. You may record any thoughts that come to you.

This is a recipe for general cleansing and uplifting bath

dash of hyssop

dash of lavender

dash of frankincense oil

dash of Florida water or clear rum

1 clear quartz crystal

1 cup of Epsom salt

Mix well in a large natural container

burn sage or frankincense and a white candle while bathing

pray or chant for clarity, peace, healing, releasing, etc.

Spiritual baths can be done one at a time, in a series of 3, 5, 7 or more days. They can be done weekly , bi-monthly or monthly depending on your need. Let your spirit guide.

The Ancient Ones were masters of energy and were able to project themselves as well as other objects through space and time. They knew how to manipulate energy and the forces around them and were able to create everything they could conceive. You also have the ability to do the same and it is important that you learn to do this at this time we are living in right now. Everything is created first by a thought, then it is spoken then it becomes manifest in the physical realm. That is how energy flows to create everything. You have to be aware and in control of your thoughts, your words and actions. Your fears can become your reality if given too much energy. It is the same for your dreams, you can have everything your really want and need when you overstand your energy and how to use it.

THE AURA

The Aura is a life sustaining energy field that surrounds every living thing. It is composed of electromagnetic radiations and affects or can be affected by our emotional, mental, physical and spiritual bodies. If it is strong it acts as a protective shield around us, deflecting negative energy from interacting with you. It should keep you away from things that are not good for you as well as keep things that are not good for you, away from you.

If your aura is weak, it will allow the penetration of other energy affect your energy, your thoughts, your actions, etc. A weak aura can have holes, tears or another persons energy clinging to it which will also affect your sekhem, your vitality, how your feel and move. If one has good character the aura is usually strong and brightly colored. If not ones negative behavior and energy tends to attract more negative energy and radiates a cloudy, dull aura. RA SEKHI is used to clear and strengthen the aura. Spiritual baths also assist in keeping the aura clear. There are many other things that can be done to keep the aura strong, see following list.

Negatively affects aura	Positively affects aura
Poor diet	Eating fresh fruits and veggies
Lack of exercise	Exercise 3-4 times a week
Lack of fresh air	Spend time outside in nature
Lack of rest	Take time to rest yourself
Stress	Meditate
Alcohol	Do positive affirmations
Drugs	Read spiritual books
Violence/ conflict	Stay around positive people
Negative habits	Take Spiritual baths
Improper psychic activity	Live with good character
Negative thinking	Laugh often
Negative environment	

The aura is colored because it is an energetic field and colors have an energetic vibration as well. Energy carries colors from infra red to ultra violet. The infra red part of the spectrum, which vibrates on a lower frequency is related to functions of the body. High frequency colors blue, indigo and purple are related to thinking creativity, intentions, sense of humor and emotions. The color or colors of your aura reflect the energy and thoughts that your have within. Some have the ability to see the colors of ones aura. With practice this gift like all psychic powers can be developed with time.

EXERCISE TO FEEL THE AURA

Press the center of your right palm and tips of fingers with your left thumb. Repeat this in left palm and fingers with your right thumb. Keep your hands a foot apart with palms facing inside. Close your eyes and slowly bring your hands close to each other and again take them apart slowly. Do this exercise a few times. The pressure of heaviness you feel is your aura.

Keep your hands a foot away from your body and slowly bring your hand closer toward the body. Repeat this a few times and you will feel your auric energy.

ARITU/ KARA KASA

We have concentrated areas of energy within us called Kara kasa, aritu, Souls of RA, chakras. The word chakra comes from the kemetic words kara which means shrine, karkar which means cylinder and thesu/kasu which means knots. The seven knots, or seven vertebre, are associated with seven Neteru who work thru these centers. These energy centers connect us to the higher forces or are aspects of the Higher Forces within us. They are connected to planets and days of the week as well.

One of the many textual references regarding the seven thesu (knots) can be found in Chapter 71 of the Pert em Hru (misnomered Egyptian Book of the Dead) scribed over *3,600 years ago:*

"...O you seven knots, the arms of the balance on that night of setting the Sacred Eye in order, who cut off heads, who sever necks, who take away hearts, who make a slaughter in the Is-land of Fire: I know you, I know your names; may you know me just as I know your names; if I reach you, may you reach me; if you live through me, may I live through you; may you make me to flourish with what is in your hands, the staff [spine]which is in your grasp.

Our Kemetic Ancestors where aware of these energy centers and their true properties many years ago. The colors that were associated with these centers , were also the colors associated with the deities of the Kara kasa,. This is one of the differences from the more common knowledge which was from an Indian perspective.

The word Aritu is a Kemetic word which is also used to describe the Kara Kasa, because it means wheel.

These are sacred energy centers are said to swirl in a circular motion very quickly and are seen as small wheels within us. They are points known to give and receive energy. When one's energy is high they all move simultaneously and continuously. Their rate of movement depends on one's vitality, if ones energy is high they move very quickly. If one has a low vibration they move slowly and sometimes not at all.

There are 7 major aritu located along our spine, 22 minor aritu throughout our bodies, one arit below our feet which connects us to the earth and at least 3 aritu over our head which connect us to the heavens. The aritu give, receive and store energy. It is at these points where energy is exchanged. It comes into us from food, sunlight, and air. Then from these points vital energy is sent to our organs, glands and other parts of our body. This energy is what keeps our bodies and minds working as they should. So if our life force is low on energy there is not much to be used and dis-ease begins in the physical. Many physical ailments come from a spiritual, mental or emotional issue that has not been process properly, therefore it causes a block in energy flow and creates sickness in the body to get you to pay attention and address your issues.

Remember energy can attach itself to you, your thoughts, feelings and/or your aura. You may feel a shift in energy when you aritu are out of balance. Sometimes you feel a shift in energy and are unaware of what you are really feeling. In RA SEKHI we seek to remove blockages and bring balance to the aritu to bring overall wellness to the ourselves. We use colors, sounds, crystals, symbols and palm healing to bring alignment and harmony to the aritu. Understanding more about the aritu will help you overstand how to keep them active and balanced.

The following charts give more information on aritu and their properties

RITU CHAKRAS 7 ENERGY CENTERS	SEKFKHET ROOT	TEKH SACRAL	OB SOLAR PLEXUS	KHEPERA HEART	SEKHEM THROAT	MER THIRD EYE	IKH CROWN
CENTRAL ISSUE	Survival	Sexuality Emotions	Power Will	Love Relationships	Communication	Intuition Imagination	Spiritual Connection Awareness
GOALS	Stability, trust Grounding, physical health	Fluidity, Feeling pleasure	Vitality, self esteem, purpose, strength of will	Balance, good relationships, compassion	Clarity, creativity, resonance	Physic ability, accuracy, clear vision	Wisdom, knowledge, high consciousness
SELF ORIENTATION	Self preservation	Self gratification	Self definition	Self acceptance	Self expression	Self reflection	Self knowledge
INSIGHTS	To be here / To have	To feel / To want	To act	To love and / Be loved	To speak and / Be heard	To see	To know
IDENTITY	physical	emotional	ego	social	creative	archetypal	universal

38

WEEKDAY	Monday	Friday	Tuesday	Thursday	Wednesday	Saturday	Sunday
PLANET	Earth and moon	Venus	Mars	Jupiter	Mercury	Saturn	Sun and Moon
DEITIES	AUSET, ODUA, YEMAYA, ADJUA	HET HRU, OSHUN BES, BAST AFI	HERUKHUTI OGUN, BENA, SEKHMET	HERU, SANGO, YAA MAAT	TEHUTI, ESU, ANANSI, SET, AKU	NEBTHET, ORUNMILA, NEKHEBET/ UCHAT, OYA AMEN-MEN	RA/RAAT, PTAH, NEFER ATUM, AWUSI, AUSAR
SENSE	Time	Taste	Balance	Touch	Hearing	Sight	Smell
COLOR	Red, blue, black	Orange, gold, green	Yellow, red, gold	Green, blue, red, white	Yellow, red, black	Indigo, white, black	Violet, white, black

KARA KASA/ SOULS OF RA/ARITU CHART

ARITU CHART 2

Crown
Foods: Purple fruits and veggies
Glands: Pineal, cerebral cortex, central nervous system, right eye
Stones: Amethyst, alexandrite, diamond, clear quartz

"I am that I am"

First Eye
Foods: Blue & purple fruits and veggies
Glands: pituitary, left eye, nose, ears
Stones: lapis lazuli, azurite, sodalite, quartz, sapphire

"I have clear vision"

Throat
Foods: Blue and purple fruits and veggies
Glands: Thyroid, parathyroid, hypothalamus, throat, mouth
Stones: Turquoise, blue topaz, chrysocolla, aquamarine, azurite

"I speak with love and clarity"

Heart
Foods: Green fruits and veggies
Glands: heart, thymus, circulation, arms, hands, lungs
Stones: Emerald, green & pink tourmaline, malachite, jade, aventurine, rose quartz

"I am Divine Unconditional Love"

Solar Plexus
Foods: Yellow fruits and veggies
Glands: Pancreas, adrenals, stomach, liver, gallbladder, nervous system, muscles
Stones: Citrine, topaz, amber, tigers eye, gold calcite, gold

"I am in control of my power"

Sacral
Foods: Orange fruits and veggies
Glands: ovaries, testicles, prostrate, genitals, spleen, womb, bladder
Stones: carnelian, coral, gold calcite, amber, citrine, topaz,

"I use my creativity for my highest good"

Root
Foods: Proteins, red fruits and veggies
Glands: adrenals, kidneys, spinal column, colon, legs, bones
Stones: ruby, garnet, bloodstone, red jasper, black tourmaline, obsidian, smoky quartz

"I am safe, secure and grounded"

PREPARATION FOR HEALING – ARITU EXERCISES

The healer must raise their own vibrations to connect with Divine healing energy. Before a day of healing it is good to do some form of physical exercise in the morning, as well as Ra Sekhi on self, to center and open the chakras. Some of the most powerful exercises I have seen to charge, brighten, clear and strengthen the aura and chakras are those taught in Kemetic and Kundalini Yoga. Here are some exercises that focus on breathing and spine flexibility to assist in opening the chakras also called Arit by our Ancestors.

Root: Sit on the floor on your heels. Place the hands flat on your thighs. Inhale and flex spine forward in the pelvic area, then exhale and flex backward. Repeat several times.

Sacral : Sit on the floor with your legs crossed. Grab you ankles with both hands and deeply inhale. Flex the spine forward and lift the chest, rotate the top of pelvis back. Exhale and flex spine back, pelvis moves forward. Repeat several times
Posture2: Lay back on your elbows with legs stretched in front of you. Inhale and raise legs with feet apart. Exhale and cross feet, inhale and open feet, exhale and cross again. Repeat several times.

Solar Plexus: Sit with legs crossed, grasp shoulders with fingers in front, thumbs in back. Inhale and twist to the left, exhale and twist to the right. Breathe deep and keep spine straight. Repeat several times and reverse direction.
Posture 2: Lie on back with legs together and raise the heels six inches. Raise the head and shoulders six inches, point to your toes with your fingertips with arms straight. In this position pant through your nose 30 times then relax for a count of 30. Repeat several times.

Heart: Sit with legs crossed, lock fingers in a bear grip at the heart center with elbows pointing out. Move elbows in a seesaw motions breathing deeply with the motion. Continue several times. Repeat movement while sitting on your heels to raise energy higher.

Throat: Sit with legs crossed with hands on knees. Keep arms straight, inhale, and shrug shoulders then exhale and push shoulders down. Repeat several times.

Third Eye: Sit with legs crossed lock fingers in bear grip at throat level. Inhale and hold your breath then squeeze your abdomen and push energy up. Exhale and raise your arms above your head holding the bear grip. Repeat several times.

Crown: Sit on your heels with arms stretched over your head. Interlock fingers except for two index fingers, which point straight up. Do 30 fire breaths then relax. Repeat several times.

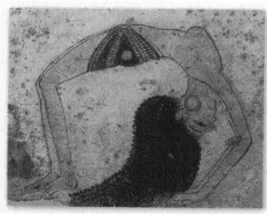

Pose of enlightenment

WORKING WITH SPIRIT GUIDES

We all have Spirit Guides who walk with us. Each of us have ancestors, (called Sheps, Egungun, Nsamafo, etc) from our direct bloodline who guide us and protect us on our journey on this realm. Some of us have other ancestors who may not be from our bloodline who assist and guide us. It is tradition to begin working with your own benevolent ancestors to strengthen and elevate their spirits. Communicating with our ancestors help to build our Ase as well as elevate and heal our entire lineage.

Ask the elders in your family about your ancestors. Write or record the stories they tell you. Share the stories with your families and friends. Make a list of your ancestors to include in your prayers. BE VERY MINDFUL OF THE ANCESTOR NAMES THAT YOU CALL. MAKE SURE TO ONLY CALL NAMES OF THOSE WHO LIVED IN A RIGHTEOUS WAY. You can learn to pour libation and create an altar space for your ancestors as well to help strengthen your connection with them.

Many of us have other Spiritual Beings (sometimes called angels) or deities who can also serve as our spirit guides. These forces , also referred to as Gods, Goddess, Neteru, Orisha, Abosom, Lwa, Loa, Nkisi, etc are seen as aspects of the All. These forces have names and attributes to help us to overstand them and nature better. As we come from the Earth and have the same elements within us that the Earth is made of, we also have these forces, the God/Goddesses forces within us as well. Some of these forces are stronger within us as individuals based of the day of the week and the date we were born. Our ancestral lineage also connects us with certain deities as well, that is why it is important to connect with your ancestors first. They will guide you to the other things about yourself that you need to know.   Those of us who are healers can have many Spirit Guides who work with us, especially during a healing session. It is important to know your spirit guides and to know how to call or invoke them to come and work with you when you need them. Spirit Guides will direct you to use the correct medicine, symbols, colors, etc. to align yourself and others. They usually speak to us with a soft subtle voice and can be seen as ones intuition. The intuition is like a gut feeling that you get, however a Spirit Guide will usually speak with direct guidance or wisdom. That first voice you hear when you are making a decision is usually your Spirit guide coming to your aid to give you direction.

You can call the presence of your Spirit Guides by pouring libation, chanting their names and praying or talking to them. You can stay connected by listening to them, make offerings or keep an altar space for them as well. You can use this libation or create your own.

Libation

Ankh (3 times)

I give thanks, honor and praises to you NTR (name that you call THE MOST HIGH). Known by many names

I salute you this day

I salute the elements Air, Fire, Water and Earth

I thank you Benevolent Ancestors, those in my lineage who lived in a righteous way I offer this water as a token of my love and blessings. (say names and pour water on the earth)

I thank you for your guidance and protection.

I thank you Great Spirit Guides, ORISA, NTRU, ABOSOM, (name Afrikan deities) who walk with me

I thank you for your presence in my life.

I thank you for your many blessings and strength.

I give thanks for my Divine Spirit and for those I am connected to.

I pray for blessings and protection for my family

I pray for blessings for my community

I pray for blessings for this world and that MAAT will be restored to the Earth once again.

I salute the animal, plant, and mineral kingdoms

And for things great and small I give thanks.

ASE AMEN RA MAAT

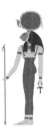

Anetch Hrak SEKHMET ,   Praises be to SEKHMET

SEKHMET is a lion headed female warrior. She is a Solar deity, known as the daughter of RA and RAAT (Infinite energy). She is the wife of Ptah (creative energy) Her name comes from Sekhem, which means powerful. She is called the Eye of RA and is seen with a solar disk and serpent crown.She is known as a fierce protector and warrior, who could heal or kill. She was worshipped mainly in upper Kemet and is known to have thousands of statues created in her honor for rituals and ceremonies. She was called on to lead the pharaohs into battle and she was called to protect the Pharaoh as well.

Working with SEKHMET is important in our practice. She is very powerful, fiery and like a lion can be gentle or very fierce. She helps us to remove toxins from our body, our homes and environment, as well as negative thinking patterns, negative habits, and all that does not serve our highest good.

She destroys ignorance and evil within one's heart. She governs and enforces divine order, plagues , epidemics, and cures. She also known as the Goddess of menstruation, the life blood which flows from women only. She works through our blood, circulatory system, heart and solar plexus. She governs our will, our drive, our vitality and motivates us to live with MAAT. She tells us that we can use all things natural to heal ourselves and will gladly assist us into bringing our lives into MAAT in all ways.

When working with her be very conscious and specific with your requests. She honors and respects good character, she is a warrior for MAAT and a fierce protector of her children. She is called the eye of RA and sees all

She has been called on through the ages to come to this plane when there is chaos on the earth. She helps to restore MAAT once again. She is the Goddess of menstruation and is associated with blood, as sekhem flows through our blood. When working with her she can cause your cycle to come, if you are a menstruating woman.   She will make you feel warm, hot or even sweat when you work with her as well.

She is associated with Tuesday, the colors red, purple and gold. Some of her favorite crystals are amethyst, citrine, carnelian, amber and bloodstone. She loves all crystals. Her favorite offerings are cherries, pomegranate, berries, watermelon, red grapes, beets, roses, rose oil, lavender or other floral oil, flowers, red wine, candles. Her herbs are ginger, garlic, red clover, and dandelion, or course. She works to heal, protect, destroy, bring justice, bring order, balance division, enhance spiritual connection, raise vitality and the like. She says we can use all things natural to heal and balance ourselves.

Following are some prayers to Invoke THE GREAT MOTHER HEALER SEKHMET.

Anetch hrak SEKHMET

Great Mother Healer

Opener of the Way

Keeper of the Divine Law

The awakener

The enlightener

Overcomer of Enemies

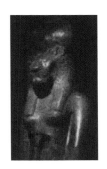

Dua SEKHMET

Thank you for healing my mind, my heart, my body and my Spirit.

Dua SEKHMET

Thank you removing all evil and toxins from within and around me.

Thank you for sharing your healing light with me and all who I am connected to.

Thank you for healing my friends, my family and community.

We ask that you restore MAAT to our lives.

We ask that you restore MAAT to the planet once again.

Destroy the wicked plots and plans that are made against your children.

Protect us from all hurt and harm.

Let us overcome our enemies.

Raise us up that we may move forward in the light of MAAT.

Dua SEKHMET

Dua NTR

ASHE AMEN RA MAAT

"Sekhmet the Powerful, powerful in her existence, She that impurity fears.

The one who's face is beautiful, remarkable of image, who thrusts back sadness.

The solar feminine disc, radiant, rejuvenating, illuminating the country.

The Mistress of the sky, appearing in her sanctuary.

Sekhmet, powerful against the enemies, inspiring terror in the rebels.

The Mistress of Inuit, entering into her chapel, whirling and dancing in her temple."

(translated into English by Kerry Wisner, 1999-2000, from the French text "Dendera – I Traduction" by S. Cauville

The Chapter of Giving a Heart to the Osiris

May the goddess Sekhmet raise me, and lift me up. Let me ascend into heaven, let that which I command be performed in Het-ka-Ptah. I know how to use my heart. I am master of my heart. I am master of my hands and arms. I am master of my legs. I have the power to do that which my KA desireth to do. My Heart-soul shall not be kept a prisoner in my body at the gates of Amentet when I would go in in peace and come forth in peace.

from the Book of Coming Forth by Day

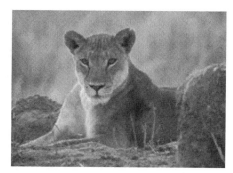

Following is a list of praise names for SEKHMET. They can be used to invoke her energy.

Sekhmet,

She Who Is Powerful

She Whose Opportunity Escapeth Her Not

Sekhmet,

Great One of Healing

Great One of Heaven

Great One of Heka

Great One of the Incense of the Ennead

Great One of Laws

Great One of Magic

Great One of the Place of Appearances in Silence

Great One of the Places of Judgment and Execution

Sekhmet,

Beloved of Ra, Her Father

Beloved of Bast, Her Sister

Beloved of Ptah, Her Husband-Brother

Sekhmet,

Ruler of the Chamber of Flames

Ruler of the Desert

Ruler of Lions

Ruler of Serpents And Of Dragons

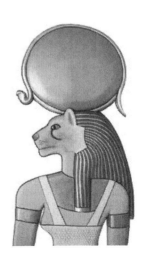

Sekhmet,

The One Who Gives Joys

The One Who Holds Back Darkness

The One Who Leads Humans

The One Who Loves Ma'at and Who Detests Evil

The One Who Presides Over the Country

The One Who Reduceth to Silence

The One Who Rouseth the People

The One Who Terrifies the Gods by Her Massacre

The One Who Terrorizes the Two Lands with Her Fear

The One Who Travels in Lightning

The One Who Was Before The Neteru Were

Sekhmet,

Lady of the Acacia

Lady of All Powers

Lady of the Bloodbath

Lady of Bright Red Linen

Lady of Darkness

Lady of Enchantments

Lady of Flame

Lady of Heaven

Lady of the House Of Books

Lady of the House of Life

Lady of Humanity

Lady of Intoxications

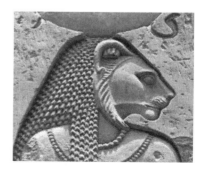

Sekhmet,

At Whose Wish The Arts Were Born

Awakener

Beautiful Eye Which Giveth Life To The Two Lands

Beautiful Face, Image Most Beloved By Art

Beloved Teacher

Bright Flame

Comforter

Destroyer By Fire

Destroyer By Plagues

Empowerer

Enlightener

Eternal As Her Father

Great Serpent On The Head Of Her Father

Guide And Protectress From The Perils Of The Underworld

Light beyond Darkness

Mightier Than the Neteru

Most Beautiful Among The Neteru

Most Strong

Praised by Her Father

Pre-Eminent in the Castle of Fire

Pre-Eminent One in the Boat of Millions of Years

Self-Contained

Sovereign

Unrivaled And Invincible One

Upholder

Victorious One In Battles

Wadjet the Great

Wanderer in the Wastes

Sekhmet,

The Aware

The Beautiful Light

The Great Defender

The One Before Whom Evil Trembles

The Source of Power

The Uraeus Who Opens the Acacia Tree

Sekhmet of the Knives

Burner of Evildoers

Destroyer of Rebellions

Eater of Flame

Eldest of Her Creator

Eye of Ra

Eye of Heru

Giver of Ecstasies

Inspirer of Men

Mistress of Ankhtawy

Mistress of the Crowns

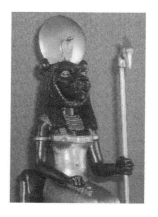

Mistress of Dread

Mistress of Enchantments

Mistress of the Two Lands

Mixture of the Night

Mother of the Dead

Mother of Images

Mother of the Neteru

Opener of Ways

Overcomer of All Enemies

Overthrower of Qetu

Protectress of The Divine Order

Protectress of the Neteru

Powerful of Heart

Queen of the Venerable Ones

Queen of the Wastelands

Roamer of Deserts

Satisfier of Desires

Shining of Countenance

Smiter of the Nubians

Sovereign of Ra

Sekhmet the Great!

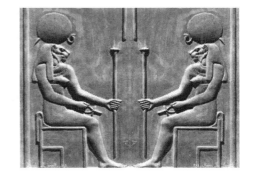

THE EMERGENCE OF SEKHMET

Excerpt from the Book of the Heavenly Cow. Found in the tombs of Tut Ankh Amen, Seti and Ra Messu

[In the language of Kamit, Ntoro (God) and Ntorot (Goddess), plural Ntorou and Ntorotu, are the Divine Spirit Forces in Creation.]

Ra (rah') is the Creator, the Ntoro (God) Who brought Himself into being. It happened that after He had assumed the sovereignty over men and women, Ntorotu and Ntorou (Goddess and Gods) and Creation, certain men and women were speaking words of complaint against Uati [The Unique One - Ra], saying:

"Look, His Majesty (Life, Strength, Health) has grown old. His bones have become like silver, His members like gold and His hair is like real lapis-lazuli." His Majesty heard the words of complaint which these men and women were speaking. His Majesty (Life, Strength, and Health) said to those who were in his following:

"Call, bring to me my Arit [Eye]and Shu and Tefnut, Seb and Nut and the Fathers and Mothers who were with me when I was in Nu together with my Father, the Ntoro (God) Nu. Let Him bring His councilors with Him. Let them be brought together in secret, so that those men and women may not perceive them and therefore take to flight with their hearts in fear. You come with them to the Great House, and let them declare their counsel fully, for I will go to Nu into the place wherein I brought about my own existence, so let those Ntorotu and Ntorou (Goddesses and Gods) be brought to me there." Now, the Ntorotu and Ntorou were drawn up on both sides of Ra and they bowed down before His Majesty until their heads touched the ground. And the

Creator of men and women, the sovereign of the rekhit (wise men and women), spoke His words in the presence of His Father Nu, the Father of the first-born Ntorotu and Ntorou. And the Ntorotu and Ntorou spoke in the presence of His Majesty Ra, saying, "Speak to us, for we are listening to your words."

Then Ra spoke to His Father Nu, "You first-born Ntoro (God) from Whom I came into being, You Ntorotu and Ntorou (Goddesses and Gods) of ancient time, my Ancestresses and Ancestors, listen to these men and women who were created by my Arit [Eye] who are speaking words [plotting rebellion] against me. Tell me what you would do in the matter, consider this thing for me and seek out a plan for me, for I will not slay them until I have heard what you say to me concerning it."

Then the Majesty of Nu spoke to His son Ra, "You are the Ntoro (God) who is greater than He who made You. You are the Sovereign of those who were created with You. Your throne is set and the fear of You is great. Let Your Arit [Eye] go against the uaiu - those who utter blasphemies against You and are plotting to rebel against You."

And the Majesty of Ra said, "Look, they have taken to flight into the mountain lands, for their hearts are afraid because of the words which they have uttered."

Then the Ntorotu and Ntorou (Goddesses and Gods) spoke in the presence of His Majesty saying, "Let Your Arit [Eye] go forth and let Her destroy for You those who uaiu en tju [rebel in disorder/evil], for there is no Arit [Eye] whatsoever that can go before Her and resist Her when She journeys in the form of the Ntorot (Goddess) Het-Heru."

The Ntorot (Goddess) then went forth and slaughtered the men and the women who were on the mountain (desert land). And the Majesty of Ra said, "Come, come in peace Het-Heru, for the work is accomplished."

Then this Ntorot (Goddess) said, "You have made me to live, and when I sekhem na (executed power) over the rebellious men and women it was sweet to my heart"

And the Majesty of Ra said "I will execute authority over them as king and I will destroy them."

And so it happened that this Sekhmet [this powerful (sekhem) One], upon the change of night, waded about in the blood of the men and women She had slaughtered, beginning at the region of Henen Su.

Then the Majesty of Ra spoke saying, "Cry out and bring to me swift and speedy messengers who can run like the wind . . . ." and immediately messengers of this kind were brought to Him. And the Majesty of Ra spoke, "Let these messengers go to Abu, and bring to me red ochre in great numbers". And when the red ochre was brought to Him His Majesty gave it to Sektet, the Ntoro who dwells in Annu (Heliopolis) to grind [Sektet is a different Ntoro than Sekhmet].

And when the royal female attendants were bruising the grain for [making] beer, the red ochre was placed in the vessels which were to hold the beer and this red ochre and beer mixture appeared to be the same color and texture of the blood of the men and women who had been slain. They made seven thousand vessels of this beer with red ochre mixture. Now, when the Majesty of Ra, the King of the South and North, had come with the Ntorotu and Ntorou (Goddesses and Gods) to look at the vessels of the beer the daylight had appeared after the slaughter of men and women by the Ntorot Sekhmet in their season. As She sailed up the river, the Majesty of Ra said, "It is good, it is good, nevertheless I must protect [the other/good] men and women from Her."

And Ra said, "Let them take up the vases and carry them to the place where the [rebellious] men and women were slaughtered by Her." Then the Majesty of the King of the South and North in the beauties of the night caused to be poured out these vases of sleep-causing beer. And the meadows of the Four Heavens were filled with water mixed with the sleep-causing beer, by reason of the Souls of the Majesty of this Ntoro (God). And so it happened that when this Ntorot (Goddess) arrived at the dawn of the following day, She found the Heavens flooded and She was pleased and she drank believing the water to be mixed with the blood of the men and women. Her heart rejoiced, however, She then became inebriated and sleepy and She gave no further attention to the remaining men and women. [Her further wrath had now been averted.]

Then said the Majesty of Ra to this Ntorot (Goddess), "Come in peace, come in peace, Amit [Amit means the Beautiful, Gracious One and the Patient One – Ra is invoking Sekhmet's patience]," and thus beautiful women came into being in the city of Aamut. And the Majesty of Ra spoke concerning this Ntorot, "Let there be made for Her vessels of the beer which produces sleep at every sacred time and season of the year and they should be in number according to the number of my royal female attendants". And from that early time until now men and women, on the occasions of the festival of Het Heru, have made vessels of the beer which make them to sleep in number according to the number of the royal female attendants of Ra.

...And the Majesty of Ra said to this Ntorot, "A feeling of the heat of melancholy has come over me. From where does this feeling come"? The Majesty of Ra said, "I live, but my heart hath become exceedingly weary with existence with them (i.e., with disordered men and women). I have slain [some of] them, but there is a remnant of worthless ones, for the destruction

which I exacted upon them was not as great as my power...."
The Ntorotu and Ntorou who were in His following responded,
"Dwell not in your weariness of them, for the power you exer-
cised over them was according to your will"...

The Majesty of this Ntoro (Ra) then said to the Majesty of Nu,
"My body longs for a return to the Original condition as in the
First Time. I will not come to another end." [Ra is weary of His
present position of ruling Creation as King from Earth and desires to return to ruling Creation as King in the Heavens – as it
was in Sep Tepi the First Time – the dawn of the Creation of
the Universe].

And so the Majesty of Nu said, "(My) grandson Shu, your eye
will serve your Father Ra as protection. (My) granddaughter
Nut, place Him [Ra] upon your back."

The Heavenly Ntorot Nut replied, "But how, my father Nu?"...
And so Nut took the form of the Divine Cow in the Heavens.
Then the Majesty of Ra placed Himself upon Her back.

The Sky Ntorot Nut after taking the form of the Divine Cow. Nut
surrounds the Earth and the stars can be found within Her
heavenly body at night. As a Divine Cow in the Night Sky/Nut
Sky, the milk from Her udders (starlight of the milky way) nour-
ishes us on Earth.

And when these things had been done, [the good] men and
women saw the Ntoro Ra upon the back of Nut [the Ntorot in
the Sky in the form of the Divine Cow]. Then these men and
women said, "Remain with us, and we will overthrow your enemies who speak words of blasphemy and plot rebellion against
you and we will destroy them."

Then His Majesty set out for the Great House and the Ntorotu and Ntorou who were in the following of Ra remained with them (i.e., with the good men and women). During that time the Earth was in darkness. When the Earth became light again and the morning had dawned, the men and women came forth with their bows and their weapons and they set their arms in motion to kill the enemies of Ra.

Then said the Majesty of this Ntoro Ra, "Your acts of violence are placed behind you, for the slaughtering of the enemies is above the slaughter [of sacrifice]" …

RA – Creator of the Universe RAIT – Creatress of the Universe

Ra and Rait (rah-ette') are the Creator and Creatress of the Universe. They function Together under the orders of Amenet and Amen - The Great Mother and Great Father Supreme Being. The Red Aten (Sun) disk surrounded by the Cobra on the Head of Ra is the Arit (Eye) of Ra from which Sekhmet came forth. The Aten and Aah (Sun and Moon) are often called the Right and Left Eyes of Ra.

There are a number of important aspects to this story. We will only focus on a few in this article. The Ntorot (Goddess) Sekhmet is also referred to as Het-Heru as well as the Arit Ra or Eye of Ra. She is sent out by Ra to destroy those who were projecting disorder into the Creative Power (uttering words/ vibrations of complaint/blasphemy – plotting rebellion). They were disrespecting Ra, meaning that they were engaged in an attempt to corrupt the Life-Force Energy of Creation that all created entities share. If they were able to pollute the Life-Force Energy, then those Afurakanu/Afuraitkaitnut (Africans) who were not engaged in such acts would still suffer. This is similar to a small group of individuals polluting the air that we all share, therefore making us all suffer.

Sekhmet goes out and kills the disordered men and women and enjoys it so much so that She states that overpowering them was 'sweet to Her heart'. She then began to wade in their blood. We must understand that in relation to the body, the immune system cells do not have a group of immune system veins to operate through. They operate through the circulatory system's veins – they 'wade through the blood' – in order to kill cancerous (rebellious) cells. Sekhmet operates as the Divine Lymphatic System, the Feminine Complement/Aspect of the Divine Immune System of Creation operant within the Divine Body of Amenet-Amen – the Great Mother and Great Father Who Together comprise the Supreme Being. [Amenet-Amen are the Supreme Being, while Ra and Rait are the Creator and Creatress Who Together proceed from Amenet-Amen to Create the Universe].

In the end, those men and women who came out to fight and to kill for Ra were honored/blessed by Him. He tells them that their acts of violence on His behalf are put behind them. Their move to kill the enemies of Ra, have thereby been given Divine sanction. While the killing of fellow citizens would normally be classified as criminal, killing the enemy in order to uphold Divine Order is given Divine sanction.

It is important to note that Sekhmet and Het Heru are Two separate and distinct Ntorotu (Deities). Sekhmet is named after Het Heru because of inherited attributes. An Afuraitkaitnit (African) female child may be given a praise-name (nickname) or middle name which is the name of her maternal aunt because she carries the same matricircular (matrilineal) clan blood (genetics), energy and characteristics of her maternal aunt. In the same fashion, the energy of Sekhmet and that of Her Elderess Het Heru is born of the matricircular clan of Rait. Thus, Sekhmet, Het Heru and other Ntorotu in this circulage (lineage) carry the title and function Arit Ra or Eye of Ra. It is also critical to understand that Sekhmet, Het Heru, Rait, Ra as well as all of the Ntorotu/Ntorou (Netertu/Neteru - Goddesses and Gods) are accessible to and communicate with Afurakanu/Afuraitkaitnut (Africans~Black People) only. They have never and will never communicate with the whites and their offspring - all white europeans, white americans, white asians, white latinos/latinas, white arabs, white hindus, white pseudo-"native" americans, etc.

Sekhmet (left) is depicted as a Lioness while Het Heru (right) is depicted as a Cow or a Female with Cow's Horns

In Aamu (region of contemporary kom el hisn), the Per Aa Sen Usarit the First (Pharaoh Senwosret I) built a temple for Sekhmet-Het Heru over 4,000 years ago. Sekhmet and Het Heru were both worshipped at this temple.

Sen Usarit - Second ruler of the 12th Dynasty in Kamit

©Copyright by Odwirafo Kwesi Ra Nehem Ptah Akhan, 13007, 13012 (2007, 2012).

For more information on Sekhmet (Abenaa in Akan) see our articles and our website:

www.odwirafo.com

Queen Sekhmet, Dread Lioness of Khem(Egypt), She who must be obeyed, the All Conquering Queen of Ethiopia By Jide Uwechia

In the Kushitic/Khemitic cosmology, Sekhmet (also spelt Sachmet, Sakhet, and Sakhmet; Greek name: Sacmis), was the primodial war goddess. Her name suited her function, and means "the Conquering Lady" or (one who is) powerful, and she was also given titles such as (One) Before Whom Evil Trembles, and Lady of Slaughter. Sekhmet was also known as the Scarlet Lady, (a reference to blood) and the Avenger of Wrongs. As the one who destroyed the evil relentlessly whilst protecting goodness she was hailed as Nyabinghi, in the upper sections of the Nile, near the borders of Southern Sudan and Uganda, ancient Ethiopia Kush the land of the first Pharaohs. Sekhmet was She who protected the nation and the Pharaoh in peace and in war. In wars the protection and strength of the Conquering Queen Mother of Ethiopia were the hopes of the Pharaohs, and in peace She was believed to stalk the land, destroying the enemies of the Pharaoh with arrows of fire.

Indeed it was said that death and destruction of the wicked and the oppressors were balsam for her heart, and hot desert winds were believed to be her breath. The protection of the Pharaohs was such a crucial function in those time as the institution was the source of all the tradition and stability of Kush and Khem. The Pharaoh – the Great Black House – was the government of Egypt, the very soul and center of all the Black-Brown people of Africa. It comprised of the King of Kush and Egypt and the college of priestly scientists, administrators, legislators and justices that guided and directed Black Africa. This establishment governed Egypt for more than 3,000 years of its recorded existence and it was the key to its stability and longevity. The Pharaoh was the source of justice, morality and righteousness. The office of the King and Queen in the Pharaoh (the great Black House) was seen as the embodiment of the energy of the Sun...Ras. The king of Egypt was verily the living son of the great God amongst men. As such it was crucial that the crucible of order and meaning be protected at all times. And this was the key function of Sekhmet the Conquering Queen Mother of Ethiopia. She was the mother and the protector of God!

The devotion of motherhood was also an aspect attributed to the Conquering Mother of Ethiopia, Sekhmet. She was viewed as a form of Hathor the primeval mother of humanity and the gods. As Hathor, she was seen as Atum's mother. Since Atum was but another name or aspect of the Kushitic/Khemitic God Amen, Sekhmet was also conceptualized as the mother of God. In particular, she was seen as the mother of Nefertum, the youthful form of Atum, and so was said to have been Ptah's lover. Ptah was the archetypal God and Nefertum's father. Sekhmet, Ptah and Nefertum were thus the original triad of Gods, worshipped especially in the ancient Egyptian city of Memphis. Sekhmet was the incarnation of the fearless lioness. She was the essence of the majesty, royalty, and power of the fierce lioness. In art, she was depicted as such, or as a shoulder length dread locks African woman with the head of a lioness, dressed in red, the colour of blood. Given that lions were her totemic animals, tame lions were kept in temples dedicated to Sekhmet like the ones in the ancient Egyptian city of Leontopolis.

The cult of Sekhmet the Powerful Dread Lady of the south was and remains widespread in Africa and in the diaspora. Sekhmet was known by different names at different time in different areas in Africa. But her core role, function and attributes remained resiliently unaltered inspite of several local embellishments. Sometimes, her identity was composited in the identity of a great ancestral female matriarch, and it was rationalized that Sekhmet had incarnated amongst humanity as that female matriarch. In the animal kingdom Sekhmet ruled as the all powerful dread lock lioness and in the human kingdom she ruled as the Queen of Queens of Kush and Khem. She was said to manifest in the physical world cyclically either as the lioness, her favorite totem or as the incarnation of an all powerful African Empress. It is usually in the human form as an African Queen that Sekhmet prefers to leave her marks on humanity. In parts of Africa where there one finds strong strains of ancient Ethiopian-Egyptian culture one finds Sekhmet composited with various localized strong women such as the Queen of Sheba and Queen Judith in ancient Ethiopia, Queen Amina in Zaira, Nigeria, Queen Kahina, the Black African Jewish Queen of the Berbers, Queen Moremi in the ancient Oyo Empire in Nigeria, Queen Idia in the ancient Benin Empire in Nigeria, Queen Ojedi among the Onitsha Igbos of Nigeria, Queen Nzinga in Angola, and Queen Nyabinghi Muhumusa of Uganda.

Origin Of Sekhmet The Egyptian mythology teaches that in the golden age of the world that Ra (also Ras) himself the king and the father of the gods ruled Egypt himself. This was the greatest age that Egypt had ever known and until the very end it was described as the age of perfection. Ra ruled for so long in that time that men forgot the number of years he had been on the throne. Eventually, even Ra got old, "for it was decreed that no man should rule forever and he had made himself man to live on earth and rule over Ethiopian and Egypt. In his oldage, "his bones were like silver, his flesh like gold and his hair like lapis lazuli." Due to the onset of senility Ras was no more an effective fighter against Apophis the Dragon of Evil, who had subsequently grown bolder in his malfeasance and "sought ever to devour all that was good and bright and kissed by the sun." Presently the evil of Apophis entered into the soul of the ancient Africans and many of them rebelled against Ras and did evil in his sight and disrespected his works. So Ras gathered the high Gods in high council, and he sent for the four living creatures that stand before his throne, Shu and Tefnut, Geb and Nut, and finally he sent for Nun the essence of the waters. Before this high and mighty council Ras made his interdiction against men, and he sought to pronounce a malediction against them for their evil, dirty, unrighteous and disrespectful ways. But Nun, speaking on behalf of the other Gods urged restraint. Because the unconstrained wrath of Rastafari could burn up the earth in totality, consuming the deserving with the undeserving. So Nun speaking for the Gods called forth and surely, for the appointment of one enthusiastic and steadfast, one burning with sincere love and devotion for the majesty of the dynasty of Ras, one commited to the regency and hegemony of the righteous Empire, to arise and defend the integrity, and the solemnity, and the sanctity and the honour of the law and the works of Ra. For as Nun argued, "if you send forth the burning glance of your eye to slay mankind, it will turn the land of Ithiopia and the entire world with it into a desert. Therefore make a power that will smite men and women only; send out that which will burn the evil but not harm the good. Send out Nyabinghi!" Then Ras consented with the urging of the Gods. "I will not send my burning glance upon the Africa, instead I will send my mother, my protector, the love of my heart to protect my holy works. I will send Nyabinghi."

Even as he spoke, Sekhmet the dread lioness, the mighty lady of Africa, "She" who must be obeyed, sprang into being. Nyabinghi, away she sped into Africa, tearing through Egypt, Ethiopia, Punt, Asmara, Mocambique, even unto Azania in the South. She slaughtered and devoured mankind until the Nile and the Niger ran red with blood and the earth besides it became desolate. Before long the most wicked among men had been slain by the Sekhmet, the dread lioness mother of Ras, Queen of Queens of Africa, and the rest prayed to Ras for mercy. And Ra spared them. Ra spared them because he wished to spare this ungrateful humanity and grant them any indulgences for which he finds an excuse. Also it is said some in places, that "Ras wished to spare them (humanity) for he hath no desire to slay all of mankind, and leave himself the ruler of a desolate and barren earth, with no human to sing and play with him. Since then until this moment, even unto tomorrow, the name and the essence of the lion goddess has lived with us, and will live with us, without any depletion of her sheer leonine potency. Sekhmet, the Majestic Lady of power, She who must be obeyed, the dread lioness goddess of ancient and modern Africa, still lives dishing out judgement and fire, through word, sound and powerful action, to those who hate righteousness, to those who hate Jah, regardless of the colour of their skin.

Jide Uwechia January 28, 2007

THE USE OF COLOR IN RA SEKHI HEALING

Colors have been used traditionally in healing, because their energy vibrates at different frequencies. The color vibrations affect our energy on different levels and can be powerful tools in energy healing. Practice color visualizations by closing your eyes and picturing yourself surrounded in different colors. Notice how different colors can change your mood or feelings. Practice color breathing by taking in different colors through your nose and/or mouth. Notice the changes in the mood and emotions. You can also use colored candles, crystals, and pieces of material as healing tools. These are some of the most commonly used colors in Ra Sekhi healing, but all colors can be used depending on the situation. Always follow and trust your Spirit and Spirit Guides to tell you what is needed.

Black is used for grounding, stability and to protect against negative energy. It contains all the colors in the spectrum. It helps to balance the root arit and can enhance one's spiritual connection, astral travel, intuition, etc.

White is known for purification, blessings, complete unity and harmony with the universe. White includes all colors of the spectrum. It represents the source of conscious creation. It will purify the body on the highest level. It will bring peace and comfort on the highest level. It blocks negativity, brings clarity and coolness, enhances clairvoyance.

Blue is the color of truth, serenity and harmony. Blue is good for cooling, calming, reconstruction, and protecting, blue will help feverish conditions, it will help stop bleeding and will help with nervous conditions. It is very good for burns and soothing the mind.   Blue is the color associated with the Great Mothers, spiritual integrity and the Sacred Heart. Electric Blue is known to protect against psychic attack and negative energy.

Green is the color of emotional healing and traveling back in time. It will balance the emotions and brings feelings of calmness and grounding. It stimulates growth and is good for healing broken bones and tissue damage. Green can be placed around family members who are ill and promotes general healing.

Yellow is the color of intellect and is used for metal stimulation. It will help you think quicker and will bring clarity of thought. It is a color associated with the ancestors and the sun, so it is powerful for spiritual upliftment and activation. It is associated with success and fighting against sorcery.

Red is used to activate healing, and to purify with heat. It should be used in small doses because it is very powerful and can be too strong for some people Red is associated with the warriors. It is energizing, rejuvenating, stimulating and fiery. Used for working the nature of the spirit.

Gold is the strongest color to help cure all illness. It is so strong that many people are not able to tolerate it, so people have to be conditioned to gold over a period of time. Gold strengthens the body and Spirit. It is the color of mastership. It represents a quantum leap in linking the physical brain and the cognitive process to the universal consciousness.

Purple will help one connect with Divine Spirit. It is good for mental and nervous problems. It helps with pain, and is used in deep tissue work. It helps heal bones and will charge you with the light of Divine freedom. It is associated with healing, spiritual reinforcement, royalty and feminine protection. Magenta is helpful for manifesting things.

RA SEKHI HAND POSITIONS

We have powerful aritu in the center of our hands. These centers can be used to give and receive energy. We use our hands as healing tools to balance and activate our energy. Before working on yourself make sure to set your healing space with incense, candle, soft music, etc. The space should be physically clean as well. Do some breathing exercises to center yourself. Pray to and call on your Spirit Guides for assistance. Rub you hands together to activate your sekhem, then you may begin.

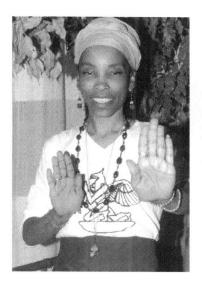 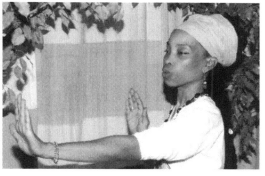

One of the first hand positions we use is called the DUA POSE. It is used to give and receive energy. Left hand and foot are always forward to stamp out negativity. It is also used in the Kemetic community as a greeting from one to another, towards an altar or a force of nature. This posture can also be done in squatting position.

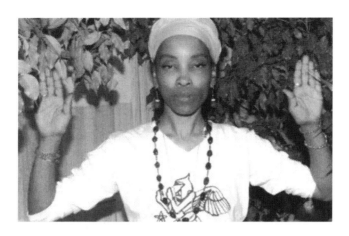

KA pose is known to assist one in connecting to the higher Spirits. It can also be used to give and receive energy.

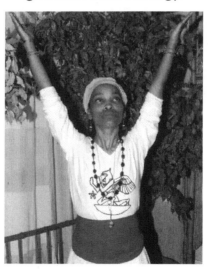

This pose its good to help one charge with the energy of RA/ RAAT and the higher forces. You will feel an extra charge when doing this while outside in the sun. Either pose is good to do while doing affirmations, chants or prayers.

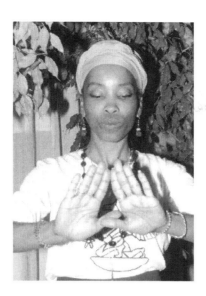

The pyramid pose is very powerful. Pyramids are associated with ancient mysteries, higher consciousness, higher knowledge, etc. When used for healing it helps to access these higher energies.

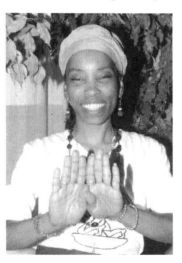 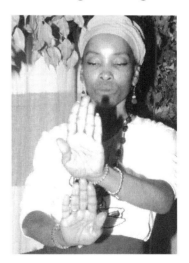

When working on self, these hand positions are used . Remember to keep your fingers together and keep your hands touching as much as possible.

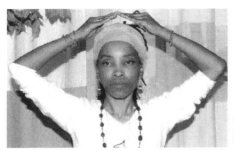

IKH CROWN ARIT

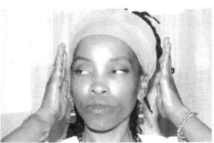

Balancing left & right hemispheres

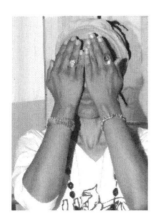

MER 1ST EYE ARIT

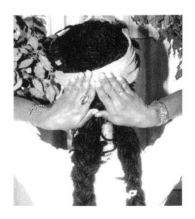

Pineal & Pituitary

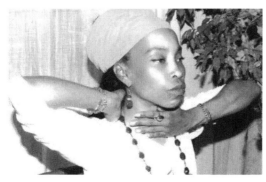

SEKHEM THROAT ARIT

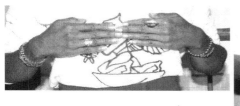
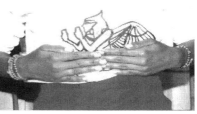

KHEPERA HEART ARIT

OB SOLAR PLEXUS ARIT

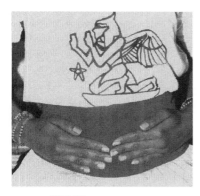
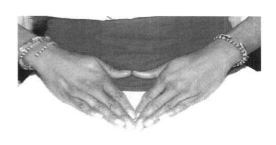

TEKH SACRAL ARIT

SEFEKHT ROOT ARIT

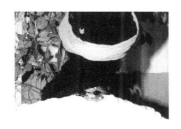
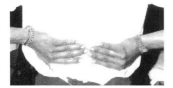
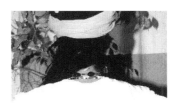
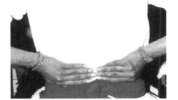

OB SOLAR PLEXUS ARIT

TEKH SACRAL ARIT

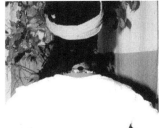

SEFEKHT root arit

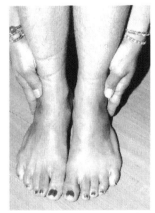

Running energy thru
aritu

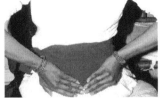

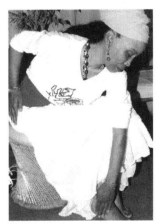

Running energy thru
legs, do both sides.

Minor arit at ankles

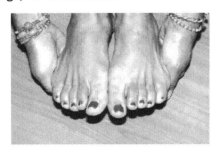

Always do center of feet
for grounding at the end
of the session

Self Treatment Healing Affirmations

POSITIONS	AFFIRMATION
HEAD	
ONE	I AM ILLUMINATION
TWO	I AM ONE WITH THE MOST HIGH
THREE	I AM AT PEACE
FOUR	I AM WORTHY, I HAVE GREAT VALUE

POSITIONS	AFFIRMATION
FRONT OF BODY	
ONE	I GIVE THANKS
TWO	I AM DIVINE & UNCINDITIONAL LOVE
THREE	I AM THAT I AM
FOUR	I AM FILLED WITH RADIANT LIGHT
FIVE	I RESPECT ALL LIVING THINGS

POSITIONS	AFFIRMATION
BACK OF THE BODY & LEGS	
ONE	I AM FILLED WITH JOY
TWO	I LOVE & ACCEPT MYSELF, I AM LOVE
THREE	I RELEASE WORRY, I AM TRUST
FOUR	I CREATE A WONDERFUL LIFE
FIVE	I AM SECURE WITH MY DIVINE SELF
SIX	I KNOW MYSELF
SEVEN	DIVINE LOVE & LIGHT LIVES & MOVES THROUGH ME

Feel free to use these affirmations or create your own.

MAJOR POSITIONS FOR SELF

	Hand position	stimulates
head	Hand over eyes	Nerves, pineal and pituitary gland
	Fingers over crown tips touching	Left and right brain and auditory system
	Hands form cradle on back of skull	Brain, pituitary, pineal and releases tension
	Hand over ears	Hearing and estuation tubes
throat	One hand over front and back of throat	Thymus, thyroid, esophagus and carotid artery
front	Fingers pointing toward each other over breasts	Heart and lungs
	One hand position down, lower rib cage	Diaphragm, liver and spleen
	One hand position lower at navel	Adrenal glands, kidneys and stomach
	One hand position lower at reproductive organs	Intestines, aorta, uterus, bladder
	Hands make pyramid finger tips at meeting place of legs	Reproductive organs
back	Hands on back of neck fingers pointing down	Vena cava, lungs, aortic arch and pulmonary arteries
	Hands over kidneys above waistline	Kidneys and adrenal glands
	Hands on mid to lower back, fingers pointing toward each other	Lower back and organs
	Fingers at base of spine forming a "V"	Coccyx and lower back

RA SEKHI SYMBOLS

We also use symbols in our practice. Symbols speak to the soul. They send messages to our subconscious and were used by our ancestors on clothes, jewelry, tailsmens, for protection, to show family ties or status, etc. The first symbols we use are symbols of the Creator/Creatress. They are universal symbols, known by many names, they represent different aspects of THE MOST HIGH, RA/RAAT, THE SUPREME BEING, LIGHT/SUN POWER, EQUALITY, HIGHER POWER, 360 DEGREES OF WISDOM, THE DIVINE ONE AND ALL.

They teach us to focus and balance the right and left hemispheres of the brain. They help to stimulate our inner power and connect with intuitive group thinking or the universal consciousness. They can be used for healing and for spiritual protection on individuals and in your environment.

The circle represent the infinite and continuous cycle of life. It has no beginning and no ending. It is associated with self, health and love. There are no limits when working with this symbol, it can be used for protection, manifesting, clarity, enhancing psychic power and the ability to focus.

The cross represents the protection. It is associated with home and community. The crossroads are known to be the meeting place or a place of making decisions. The equal cross can also be used as a cube. It is good for protection, clarity, opportunity, wisdom.

The triangle is associated with family, vitality, creation, ancient mysteries and opening the way. It is associated with the pyramid shape. Seen as God the Creator God the Giver and God the Sustainer. It is activating and fiery and can be useful in manifesting, projections, astral travel and ancestral work.

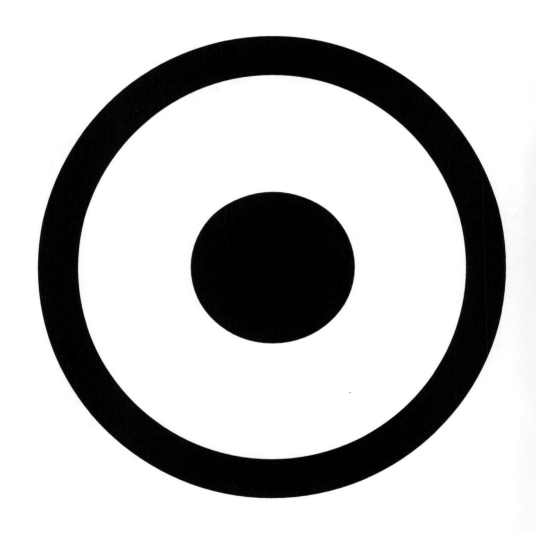

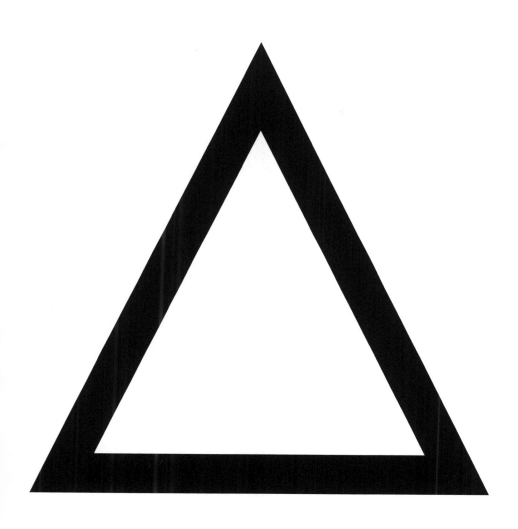

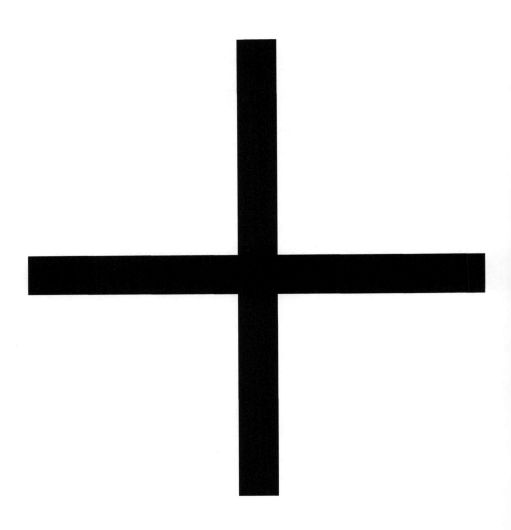

RA SEKHI SPIRITUAL PRINCIPLES

I AM THAT I AM

I GIVE THANKS FOR MY MANY BLESSINGS

I AM FULL OF LOVE, JOY, HARMONY, GOOD HEALTH AND ABUNDANCE

I AM FREE OF ANGER, WORRY, DOUBT, SAD-NESS, AND FEAR

I HAVE ALL THAT I NEED AND MORE

I SHARE LOVING THOUGHTS, WORDS AND AC-TIONS WITH ALL LIVING THINGS

I HONOR MY CREATOR, MY ANCESTORS, PAR-ENTS, TEACHERS AND MYSELF

I CLAIM HEALING FOR MYSELF, MY FAMILY, MY PEOPLE AND THE WORLD

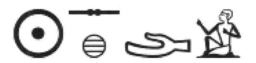

" Remember to spend a few minutes every day working with the spiritual principles of RA SEKHI.

" Apply the RA SEKHI hand positions and pronounce them with intent while giving yourself a RA SEKHI treatment. to etch the principles into your body.

" Take a long, deep sighing breath after saying each principle aloud; you are doing trauma release as you are etching the principles into your body and mind.

" As you continue to work with these principles, work on your own affirmations and principles.

" These exercises turns the Spiritual Principles of RA SEKHI into spiritual practice rather than just and recitation of a simple pledge or oath.

" When you are pouring RA SEKHI energy into the principles, they become manifestation statements. They will produce physical, mental, emotional, and spiritual changes in your mind, body, and spirit.

The Work

The information we have shared is the foundation for shifting your lifestyle to incorporate the ancient techniques of our ancestors to make our lives better. These are basic tools you can use daily to maintain overall good health and wellness. However they will not work for you by just reading the words. You have to do the work, to clear your aura, activate your aritu and maintain a high vibration. Set a time for yourself to focus on your healing. Take 21 days to do a colon cleanse, take blood cleansing herbs, fast (raw food fast) for 3– 21 days, do full body work on yourself everyday, recite laws of MAAT everyday, pour libation to ancestors everyday, do a spiritual bath for 3-7 days, do exercise to activate your aritu everyday, and drink plenty of water.

This will charge you and set your vibration at a very high level. The goal is to clear negative energy from your mental, spiritual, emotional and physical bodies. Your intuition will increase, your senses will become stronger, other spiritual gifts will develop or be enhanced, you will begin to think and feel better, etc. Then you must continue the work to maintain your vibration and culti- vate your sekhem even more. You can always take it to a high- er level. These changes do not happen overnight however the energy you put into it will determine what you receive and what changes occur. You have to focus on the work if you want it to work for you.

Here are some tips to using the tools:

* Do spiritual baths regularly, once or twice a week

* Work with your ancestors daily, change the water on your altar everyday, leave a small offering and sit with them sev- eral times a week

* Do chakra exercises or other exercise 3-4 times a week

* Work on yourself daily

* Do affirmations daily

* Do conscious breathing daily

* Call on The Great Mother Healer Sekhmet on Tuesdays, Thursdays, Fri days and Sundays

* Recite the laws of MAAT daily

* Set a morning ritual/ schedule for your practice, you can do it before your family wakes up or include them in your ritual

* Hang the symbols up in your room so you can see them and focus on them everyday

* Begin to dress and eat by the color of the day to be more in tune

* Use colors and symbols while you work on yourself, visualize them surrounding and filling your body

* Spend more time developing your spirit and cultivating sekhem (less time watching TV)

* Make the time to work on yourself, it is a priority

* Learn more about living healthy, herbs, healing, etc.

* Resolve and let go of trauma and issues of the past

The work of healing the self is continuous. I still work on myself on a regular basis. This work will not allow you to escape life, you will still have challenges, that is a part of our experience on earth. However, using these tools will allow you to face and get through the challenges better. Remember you have to use the tools for them to work for you.

ASCENSION

Ascension is about learning the lessons, laws, and truths in life and then using that knowledge to manifest your best, highest self. It about being able to look at your own mistakes as well as those of others and make a conscious choice to do the

GODLY/ MAATIC thing. Ascension is about raising your vibration, your sekhem, to fight the temptations in life and to stay in alignment with that which is right. Wherever you are you can make a conscious choice to ascend. To live with unconditional love, to live righteously, to do what is best for yourself and others. To ascend is to take care of yourself, take care of your body temple, your mind, and your heart.

Ascension is about manifesting yourself as one with THE CREATOR in thought, word and deed. Its about realizing you are free to be the CREATOR OF YOUR LIFE. Ascension is finding peace within that is so strong that nothing shakes it. It is realizing your mission and living it.

An initiation is a process or ritual which takes you from one level of consciousness to a higher level of consciousness. After the initiation, practice, work, dedication, fortitude, patience, lessons, experience, and sacrifice you exert will determine your process of ascension. Initiation is a declaration to the universe that you will actively work on your spiritual evolution.

Sacrifice is the giving of something of value to receive something of greater value in the future. Sacrifice is made in all initiations, there must be some giving of self in order to receive the blessings from the Spirit Realm. In this case, your fast and weekend in the bush is seen. Though there may be further sacrifice necessary for you to achieve your highest heights. More than anything physical you can give or do for yourself or the Higher Spirits, your time and energy to the work is the greatest sacrifice or offering you can make.

Ascension is processing all that you have learned and living it to uplift your self, and your people and to leave the world in a better place than it was before you came here.

Will you do what it takes to ascend?

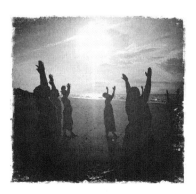

Testimonies

I am a Nubian male who has just finished Ra Sekhi level 1. I had doubts coming into Ra Sekhi, the doubt was not about the program but if it would really help to develop me in my spiritual practice. I have cleansed myself of negative energies, my spiritual senses have opened and I am more aware than I had been coming into this system of healing and the big plus for me is that the ancestors and spirit guides on the other side have spoken out to me and I have connected. I dedicate at least 2 hours a day in practicing all that was taught to me while in Ra Sekhi and I can actually feel the shift in my energy and my character. As I continue to work on myself I can only see myself getting better. The sister Nia (Kajara) is the real deal and can assist you on your spiritual path...the key is...You have to do the work! She has answers and she will help you cleanse yourself inside. Listen to your spirit if you are contemplating the classes. You will not be disappointed.

Amun RE Athan (B. Lewis)

"Ra Sekhi is the Truth. It is one of the many principles of nature/ that must be utilized to strengthen our bodies, minds and spirits. The Ra Sekhi training and private sessions I received helped me in many ways. The many clients that I have given Ra Sekhi to have come back to me with positive life changing stories that helped them to get back on track with their life's mission. God Bless our divine anointed Sister and Rhekit Kajara for waling the path of self development. Her Divine Appointment to present Ra Sekhi courses and retreats are shining example of what each and every one of us can do when we are living the principles of Maat. May every child, woman and man enter the gates to awaken their god given talents, gifts and abilities with peace, health, love, joy and abundance."

Kim Yokely Kimochi Body N Sole Sanctuary

After I received my attunement to the third level of Ra Sekhi, I noticed a drastic change in my life and in my own energy field. Everything seemed to accelerate, and I became a magnet for other light bearers as well as those desperately seeking healing. Dogs would begin to bark at me from a block away; they could feel me coming. Likewise, my ancestors and spirit guides began to speak to me much more loudly and clearly than they had before. Because of this practice, my ability to heal myself and to facilitate healing in others has been greatly multiplied. I am eternally grateful to Most High, to all of my helpful ancestors and guides, to the goddess Sekhmet, and to our beautiful teacher and founder Rekhit Kajara Assata Nebthet. May this potent energy that we are cultivating continue to evolve and be spread all across this beautiful altar we call Earth.

In loving light,
Ekua Adisa

Healing Earth's Womb

In the late 90's I found myself in a very abusive relationship. With all that was going wrong in my life, including bouts of depression I found myself having my tubes tied. I feel like I did this to get back at him for all the wrong he did to me and our children. In late December 1999 my ex husband beat my oldest son to death. He was only 4. I was to say the least in very bad shape. With no end to my grief in sight I choose to drink and smoke my problems away.

By 2004 I was floundering around trying to figure out what I wanted to do with my life. In 2005 I re-dedicated my life to a practicing Muslim. This was a first step into getting my health back on track and reconnecting to God, best thing I ever did. I'm forever grateful for The Nation of Islam and The Hon. Minister Louis Farrakhan.

Moving forward...

I always thought I would never get married again and for that matter have more children. I was done with DC and ready to move until my best friend, Enoch El Shamesh (we loved each other in High School but never dated) came back from college and convinced me not to move to Philadelphia. We married January 5th, 2010. I told my husband from the jump that I wasn't able to have anymore children, he was ok with this and told me we were still going to try.

In 2011 I had the pleasure of meeting Sister Kajara Nia Yaa Nebthet. Before meeting her I had already been attuned to Reiki energy but with her I learned the Kemetic Reiki style and learned about herbs that would benefit the healing of my womb. I've been working on myself and the healing of my womb for about a year and a half now. Recently I went to the OB/GYN and had a sonogram done. Within a weeks time I had my results from the sonogram and I was so surprised to learn that I'm now able to have children again. GIVE THANKS! GIVE THANKS! All the prayers, meditation, fasting, and good food have paid off for the better. I'm ever so grateful for all that I've been through and for what's to come. I've learned to love myself more. Love my womb more. Talk to my womb more. Be more mindful of what goes inside my body. Til next time... baby in our sights...GIVE THANKS!

Qamarah Muhammad El-Shamesh

Afterword

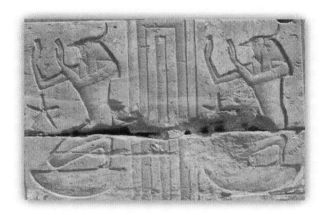

Rekhitu

*...When the scribe Ani maakheru arrives at the seventh **arit** he says: I have come to you **Ausar**, purified of disordered emanations. You encircle the heavens, you see **Ra**, you see the **Rekhitu**. Unique One, You from the **Sektet** boat - the boat of **Ra**, as He encircles the horizon in the heavens...* [**Ru Nu Pert em Hru** – Book of Coming Forth by Day, Papyrus of Ani]

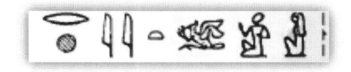

Rekhitu

The term **rekhit** in the language of Kamit (Egypt) is multi-layered in meaning. The root **rekh** means *knowledge*. **Rekhit** means *one who is wise, knowledgeable, skillful*. The **Ntorot** (**Ntrt**/ Goddess) **Auset** thus carries the title **Rekhit** meaning the *Divine Wise One* referencing Her wisdom and skill as a Divine Healeress. There exists a class of Afurakanu/Afuraitkaitnut (Africans) in ancient Kamit who are called the **rekhitu** (plural).

The **rekhitu** exist as a group within the Afurakani/Afuraitkaitnit (African) population and retain this status upon transition to the-Ancestral-realm after death. Hence, the declaration quoted above from the *Pert em Hru*. The deceased individual comes before **Ausar**, the **Ntoro** (**Ntr**/God) Who is the Sovereign of the Ancestral realm, and notes that by virtue of purification **Ausar** has taken up His position with **Ra** (Creator) in the **Sektet** boat. **Ausar** therefore encircles the heavens in this 'boat' of the **Aten** (Sun). He beholds **Ra** and also the **Rekhit** spirits. The spirit of the deceased individual endeavors to be pure and participate in the same process as **Ausar**. Moreover, in the *Emergence of Sekhmet*, it is stated that **Ra** is the "*Creator of men and women and sovereign of the rekhit.*"

The **rekhitu** are symbolized by the lapwing bird with hands raised in the act of *ritual provocation*. They are also represented in human form with the wings of the bird or as humans with the head of the bird:

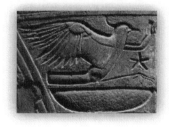

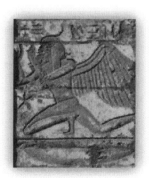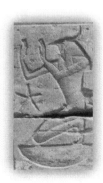

The rekhit as a sacred *Divine* bird denotes the capacity of our spirits to enter, fly, between the physical world and the spirit-realm. The upraised hands not only denote *worship*, but *ritual provocation* of the energy and consciousness of the **Ntorotu/Ntorou** and the **Aakhutu/Aakhu** – the Goddesses/Gods and the Spiritually Cultivated Ancestresses/Ancestors of Afuraka/Afuraitkait (Africa).

The **rekhit** is a spirit-medium, akin to a form of **okomfo** in Akan culture and an **elegun** in Yoruba culture. A rekhit provokes the energy and consciousness of the Ntorotu/Ntorou and Aakhutu/Aakhu by entering into communion with Them. Such communion facilitates spirit-possession of various forms. The rekhit thus becomes a *human divinatory instrument* utilized by the Ntorotu/Ntorou and Aakhutu/Aakhu for the healing and empowering of the Afurakani/Afuraitkaitnit (African) community. Their capacity to heal not only facilitates realignment of the individual from the disalignment of dis-ease. It also motivates us to re-discover our *own capacity* to heal and empower ourselves and our families through realignment with the Ntorotu/Ntorou and the Aakhutu/Aakhu Who are connected to us by blood. In this manner the community reestablishes its footing within the **sekher** (plan) of **Amenet** and **Amen**, the Great Mother and Great Father Whom Together comprise the Supreme Being.

Yet, the capacity of the rekhit to become a divinatory instrument of healing is solely dependent upon the receptivity of the rekhit to his or her **Ka/Kait** (Soul-Divine Consciousness), the **Ntorotu/Ntorou** connected to him/her and his/her **Aakhutu/Aakhu**.

Rekhit Kajara Assata Nebthet has made herself receptive and thus **Ra** and **Sekhmet** gave her **Ra Sekhi** through the agency of her Aakhutu/Aakhu (Ancestresses and Ancestors) and

Kemetic Reiki was reborn. Afurakanu/Afuraitkaitnut (Africans) as a community now benefit from her willingness to listen.

The term *reiki* is not an asian term. It is an *asian corruption* of an ancient term from Kamit. The false etymology of *rei* meaning *spiritual, natural, divine* and *ki* meaning *vital, energy, life force* is stolen from the name of **Ra**. **Ra** and **Rait** are the Creator and Creatress of the Universe. They are the *Divine Living Energy* moving throughout and animating all *created* entities. They use the **Aten** (Sun) as a physical transmitter of Their Spiritual Energy. The name **Ra** (rah) in the past and currently is consistently corrupted and mispronounced by eurasians as *Re* (rei). The term **khi** and **khai** are actually *titles* of **Ra** delineating the *exalted* nature of His *fiery* energy. Moreover, **Rekhi** is one of the 75 forms of **Ra**:

Rekhi, Tomb of Seti I, one of the 75 forms of Rā (No. 40).

The 〄 **metut** (hieroglyph) in the inscription of the name is a determinative symbol of a brazier pot with a flame referencing *fire* and *heat*.

There is no such thing as an ancient asian healing practice, for the only ancient people in existence are Afurakanu/ Afuraitkaitnut (Africans).

It is Afurakanu/Afuraitkaitnut (Africans~Black People) - **and only Afurakanu/Afuraitkaitnut** - wherever we exist in the world, who have the capacity to invoke the *Divine Spirit Forces* that govern Creation (**Ntorotu/Ntorou; Abosom; Orisha; Vodou; Arusi**) and the *Spiritually Cultivated Ancestresses and Ancestors* (**Aakhutu/Aakhu, Nananom Nsamanfo, Egungun, Kuvito, Mmuo**) for our realignment, healing and advancement.

Ra Sekhi is a conscious reconstitution of an ancient practice of **Khanit** and **Kamit** (Nubia and Egypt) that Afurakanu/Afuraitkaitnut carried with us to North, Central, South and West Afuraka/Afuraitkait after migration from the valley of **Hapi** (Nile). It is a practice we continued as Akan, Yoruba, Igbo, Ewe, Goromantche, Bakongo, Fang and all others. It is a practice that we carried with us through the **Mmusuo Kese** (the Great Perversity/enslavement). Often without access to medicinal plants as captives during enslavement, we called on the Spirits of our Nananom Nsamanfo, Egungun, Kuvito, we called on the Spirits of the Abosom, Orisha, Vodou for guidance. They directed us through dreams, spirit-possession and in the "laying of hands" to heal our people in the backwoods of Mississippi, Alabama, georgia, virginia, florida, the carolinas, maryland and elsewhere. It is this practice which we carried with us as we freed ourselves from enslavement and established independent **akofo** (warrior/warrioress – maroon) settlements after waging war against the white slavers and emerging victorious. It is this practice which we carried with us as we migrated "up north", instinctively and intuitively reestablishing shrines to our Nananom Nsamanfo and Abosom, Orisha and Egungun, Vodou and Kuvito in urban environments, cramped apartment dwellings, the backyards of our homes, in our living rooms, basements and bedrooms.

Ra Sekhi although lost by name during these times contributed to our survival. **Ra** and **Sekhmet** direct us now to fully reestablish the practice of **Ra Sekhi** as a component of communal healing which encompasses the healing of our people, the restoration of our sovereignty and the eradication of our enemies.

Odwirafo Kwesi Ra Nehem Ptah Akhan 13012 (2012).

TUA NTR

I give thanks to the Creator/Creatress. I give thanks to my Benevolent Ancestors. I give thanks to my Spirit Guides and to the GREAT MOTHER HEALER SEKHMET. I give thanks to my Mother and Father, who have always been there for me I love and honor you both. I give thanks to my youth, Nile, Yahsh, Nzi and Ori everything I do and have done is to make life better for you. I love you all unconditionally and give thanks for your patience and for sharing your Mama with many. I give thanks to my Grandmothers Christine and Nannie who showed me an example of MAAT in the flesh.

I give thanks to my teachers Queen Afua, Dr Afrika, Dr Ayaba, Grandmother Nataska Hummingbird, Ras Sekou, Sister Joyce, Sis Dorcas, El Ha Gahn, and Dr Akua.

I give thanks to my extended family those who have supported me and this healing work Ruqayyah thanks for your continuous encouragement and for being a true Sister friend. Dua Ra Nehem, my research Brother who has been there since Ra Sekhi began. Thank you for finding the proof to this work coming from Kemet and for confirming the messages I was hearing to continue to move forward with this work. Malcolm thank you for your continued love and support.

To my first students Yosafe, Aya, Shanika, Nut, Sat Ra, Stacey, Ekua, Diedra, Freedom, Queen B, Sekhmeti, I thank you for coming forth and allowing us to be a part of this healing movement together. To my Sacred Woman Sisters I love and thank you all for your energy.

To all Ra Sekhians practitioners, and initiates.....I thank you and love you all...let the healing continue.

THE POWER IS IN OUR HANDS

This book is a tool to assist with your self healing. It does not include the attunement, which is the traditional way of passing energy. We currently offer online, personal and group classes.

If you would like to register or get more info about Ra Sekhi classes and events visit us online

LEVELS OF RA SEKHI

LEVEL 1 focuses on self healing. It assists one in learning to sense and cultivate Sekhem. It allows the initiate to gain the experience of the healing system by working on self first, then family and friends. It works to develop the spiritual and mental connection using the Ra Sekhi principles. Working with the tools give the initiate a greater chance of success and support in ones spiritual development and healing.

LEVEL 2 is the Practitioner level. Once you learn to manage energy you can move on to this level. It gives the initiate more tools, energy and certification to work with other as a practitioner. These tools strengthen the healers knowledge builds concentration, ashe (spiritual power) and builds sekhem. It enhances spiritual connection, practitioners develop intuition and learn how to use a pendulum, sound therapy, and higher level of concentration and more. Distance healing, symbols , crystals, mantras, pendulums, chakra balancing, aura cleansing, spiritual protection are also a part of this level.

LEVEL 3 is the Master Teacher level for those who wish to teach RA SEKHI to others. It allows the healer the personal and spiritual development to pass Attunements and share the healing techniques with others. Purification rites for the elements air, fire, water and earth are some of the requirements to attain this level. It is also recommended that the initiate complete and practice level I and II for three to six months before attempting to move to this level.

LEVEL 4 is the Snwt or Priesthood level for those who want to work with GODDESS SEKHMET on a higher level. Only Master teachers move to this level. Training is given as a Healer Priest or Priestess and one is initiated into the priesthood of Sekhmet. Strict requirements are to be fulfilled at this level.

Level 5 is the level of Rekhit, teacher of teachers, keeper of sacred knowledge and mysteries. The amount of commitment, dedication, time, practice and energy that the Snwt gives to their work will determine the amount of time it takes to reach this level.

If you would like to host classes in your city

or attend classes with Rekhit Kajara Nebthet

Email rasekhitemple@gmail.com

or see our calendar online

www.rasekhihealing.com

Contact our certified teachers for level 1 & 2 classes, healing sessions, crystal therapy, ear candling and aura cleansing.

Atlanta GA:
Sat-Ra Sobukwe-SoDaye'
Website: www.khepraspa.com
Email: kheprahealingspa@gmail.com

Wash DC :
Qamarah Muhammad El-Shamesh
www.qamarahmoon.wix.com/qamarahs-healing-hands
Email: qamarahmoon@gmail.com

Toronto CA:
Ethereal Chanie-Margareta Sat En Hetet
Email: etherealchanie@gmail.com

Charlotte NC
Aura Agape
www.herbnspicewellness.com
Email: aurasendinluv@gmail.com

Birmingham AL
Sanovia Muhammad
Email: sanoviamu@att.net

South Bend IN
Lauren Markham
Email: LadyLo2u@yahoo.com

Oakland
Brenda Hudson
Email: Brendahudsonoo@aol.com

For Ra Sekhi healing sessions visit our Certified Practitioners

In Hartford CT:
Nefermul Mas   www.the-diamond-life.com
                       diamondlifeunlimited@gmail.com

Philly PA:
Angela Walker   hills7sea@aol.com
                       www.wallstreetphilly.com
Lonnie Davis   lonniemo@gmail.com

Wash DC:
Jazmyn Miles   jazmynmiles09@gmail.com
Maat Sekhem Akhita   ccpeeples@gmail.com

Charlotte NC:
Ifasayo   tite519@yahoo.com
Gagan Hunter   gaganjii@earthlink.net
                       www.gaganhunter.com

Long Beach CA:
Nova Kafele   Novakafele@gmail.com
                       Krstmoorproduce.spruz.com

Chicago IL:
Aya Posey   christaaya@gmail.com
Neffera Tresica Samuel   maaticembrace@yahoo.com

NY area
Robyn Mahone Lonesom   uhurabiz@earthlink.net
Tabia Beckett   yagottaloveus@gmail.com

Birmingham AL:
Demetrius Newton Jr.   Newpowrsol@bellsouth.net

Northern CA:
Tchiya Amet El Maat   amet13@tchiya.com
Cosmic Sound Healing   www.cosmic.tchiya.com

Cleavland OH
Nefer Abka Hotep   Sacred Goddess Ministries.com
                         sacredgoddessministries@gmail.com

One of our goals is to create a community that will provide a loving, learning, and caring environment for ones to come and heal from dis-eases of the body, mind, and spirit.
This community will be eco-friendly and will include the use of solar energy, organic farming and other natural resources and techniques to ensure sustainability. The community will offer events, classes, retreats natural healing products and a variety of holistic healing modalities to facilitate healing throughout the community.
We intend to create a healthy environment for children, individuals, and families to come throughout the year to learn, share, heal and experience the beauty of and reconnect with Mother Earth.

For more info and to support this vision visit
www.gofundme.com/191dl0

Visit our sister sites as well

www.youtube.com/rasekhiartstemple

www.facebook.com/rasekhiartstemple

www.niadesigns.etsy.com

www.itsnatural11.weebly.com

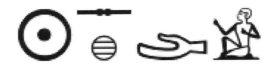

RA SEKHI ARTS TEMPLE OF HEALING

Disclaimer

RA Sekhi Arts Temple of Healing will not diagnose or attempt to cure any diseases.

Participation with RSATH is voluntary and one must accept full responsibility for the management of their own health care.

RSATH does not give a medical diagnosis, prognosis or substitute for medication or medical advice.

Made in the USA
Charleston, SC
31 January 2014